HOW TO CONTROL THE UNCONTROLLABLE

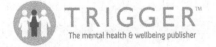

TRIGGER™
The mental health & wellbeing publisher

HOW TO CONTROL THE
UNCONTROLLABLE

ABOUT THE AUTHOR

Ben Aldridge writes about practical philosophy, comfort zones, mental health and adventure. You'll find him climbing mountains, learning Japanese, running marathons, solving Rubik's cubes, eating bizarre food, taking ice baths and sleeping in unusual places. The challenges that he sets for himself and his readers are often quirky, fun and demanding. Ben is the author of *How to Control the Uncontrollable*, *How to Be Comfortable with Being Uncomfortable* and the *Get Out of Your Comfort Zone* cards. For more information on how to connect with Ben, visit www.benaldridge.com or via his Instagram, @dothingsthatchallengeyou.

HOW TO CONTROL THE UNCONTROLLABLE

10 GAME-CHANGING IDEAS TO HELP YOU THINK LIKE A STOIC AND BUILD A RESILIENT LIFE

BEN ALDRIDGE

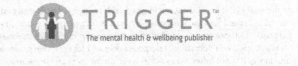

TRIGGER™
The mental health & wellbeing publisher

This edition published in 2023 by Trigger Publishing
An imprint of Shaw Callaghan Ltd

UK Office
The Stanley Building
7 Pancras Square
Kings Cross
London N1C 4AG

US Office
On Point Executive Center, Inc
3030 N Rocky Point Drive W
Suite 150
Tampa, FL 33607
www.triggerhub.org

A CIP catalogue record for this book is available upon request from the British Library
ISBN: 978-1-83796-248-8
Ebook ISBN: 978-1-83796-249-5

Typeset by Lapiz Digital Services

For Helen and Oli

CONTENTS

Introduction   xi

Part 1: Ben's Guide to Stoicism   **1**
1   What's All This Stoicism Business, Anyway?   3
2   A Brief History of Stoicism   17

Part 2: The Stoic Principles   **29**
3   Principle 1: Voluntary Discomfort   31
4   Principle 2: Perception   45
5   Principle 3: Setbacks   59
6   Principle 4: Self-reflection   73
7   Principle 5: Role Models   87
8   Principle 6: Negative Visualization   99
9   Principle 7: Managing Strong Emotions   113
10   Principle 8: Dealing with Others   127
11   Principle 9: Memento Mori   141
12   Principle 10: The Cosmic Perspective   155

Part 3: Putting Stoicism into Practice   **169**
13   Stoic Words   171
14   The Stoic Challenges   175
15   The Future of Stoicism   185
16   Upgrading Stoicism   191

Final Thoughts   197

How to Build a Stoic Library   199
The Stoic Cheat Sheet   209
Acknowledgements   215
Come and Say Hi   217

INTRODUCTION

"Just keep in mind: the more we value things outside our control, the less control we have."

Epictetus

Every single one of us will encounter tough times. There's no escape. We will all face adversity at some point. Pain, fear, grief, boredom, anger, frustration, anxiety – they are all part of our lives. This is what it means to be human. But what if there was a way to make these tough times easier? What if we could become more resilient to the challenges of life? The philosophy of Stoicism has a lot to say about this. Packed with wisdom and timeless advice, this ancient school of thought is something I wish I had known about sooner. As it happened, I had to learn the hard way ...

Several years ago I began experiencing severe and debilitating anxiety. There wasn't anything in particular that had triggered all of this – no crisis or trauma prompted it. The anxiety snuck up on me, as if out of nowhere. I started having panic attacks which felt as if I was about to die and the world might implode inside my head. It was terrifying. Imagine the adrenaline you feel before doing something scary. Now imagine that adrenaline never going away – I had this constant feeling that I was in a dangerous situation. It was relentless, exhausting and made me feel permanently on edge. I couldn't sleep. I couldn't eat properly. I felt scared all of the time. Simple things like walking to my local park and catching the bus were overwhelming and I ended up not able to leave my house.

I was so poorly educated about mental health that when I began experiencing all of these symptoms, I genuinely thought that I was dying. It felt as if I had a terminal disease and that I would soon be six feet under. I didn't understand how powerful the mind was, and I didn't think for one minute that this was a mental health issue.

The reason I mention my experience with anxiety is because it led me to discover Stoicism. In order to deal with my fear and panic attacks and better understand what was happening to me, I began reading. This wasn't casual reading, this was reading as if my life depended on it. I consumed a huge variety of books on a wide range of topics – everything from psychology to philosophy to self-help. My home became a library.

Then I discovered Stoicism. This ancient Greek philosophy resonated with me deeply and I became obsessed with it. I loved its practicality – it was a philosophy built on ideas that I could actually use. This advice was over 2,000 years old and yet still made perfect sense today.

The Stoics were resilience experts and would do crazy things to cultivate their mental strength. This particular element of Stoicism was my gateway into the philosophy. The Stoics believed that by practising adversity, you would be prepared for future adversity. I absolutely loved this concept! When I read about the Stoic philosopher Cato deliberately wearing something embarrassing to test out his mindset, I was hooked. Why would someone deliberately go out of their way to embarrass themselves? Being an introvert, the thought of this sent shivers down my spine.

I continued to learn about the Stoics and my obsession grew. I read about them exposing themselves to hardships by enduring the heat and the cold or sleeping on hard surfaces as a way to train their minds. I discovered that they would fast and "practise poverty" by wearing rough clothes and walking barefoot. This wasn't the sort of thing I associated with philosophy and it caught my attention. There were all sorts of unusual ways that the Stoics would cultivate mental resilience and I found it fascinating.

MY CHALLENGES

Inspired by these ideas, I started creating my own challenges to help me step outside of my comfort zone. This counter-intuitive method of leaning into discomfort and adversity changed everything for me and completely turned my life around. It taught me about who I was and helped me to manage my anxiety. I learned what coping mechanisms worked when I was scared and started to believe in myself again.

My personal stoic challenges were varied and tested me in several ways. Some were physical, some were mental and some were skill-based. They all pushed me outside of my comfort zone in different directions ... I ran my first marathon, climbed mountains and completed a long-distance walk. I started playing around with cold exposure – cold showers, wild swimming and ice baths. I learned how to solve a Rubik's Cube in under a minute, began studying Japanese and learned how to fold a ton of origami models. I faced a serious fear of needles by getting acupuncture, slept on the floor and wore strange things. I learned how to memorize an entire deck of cards by just looking at each card once and taught myself to pick locks. I also queued for no reason other than to test my mindset. This is just scratching the surface – there were so many ways that I pushed myself.

Seeking out challenges and difficulties changed my life. It became my go-to system of self-development. Each time I did something that I thought I couldn't, I received such a boost in confidence. It ended up being one of the most important revelations I ever made.

I wrote a book about this journey called *How to Be Comfortable with Being Uncomfortable: 43 Weird and Wonderful Ways to Build a Strong Resilient Mindset*. In the book I wrote about the challenges that helped me to build my mental resilience, and Stoicism was threaded throughout the book but it wasn't the main theme of the project.

Stoicism is such a rich philosophy, packed with so many practical ideas that it deserves a book in its own right, so that's what you're holding now. This book is my tribute to the philosophy that changed my life. It's an exploration of Stoic ideas and a chance for me to share the practical ways the philosophy has benefitted me.

Initially the philosophy helped my severe anxiety but as this got under control, the ideas started to bleed into other areas of my life. I now use Stoicism every single day. I use it when I'm doing adventurous things and not-so-adventurous things. It's helped me in wild and remote mountain settings and closer to home when dealing with obstacles and things that don't go to plan. It's helped me to manage strong emotions like anger and fear and taught me how to deal with difficult and demanding people. It was also incredibly helpful for me when dealing with the complicated and tense premature birth of my little boy, Oli. There are so many things that this philosophy has helped me with.

Everything I write about in this book comes from self-study and practical application – essentially me testing stuff out in the real world. The concepts in these pages are the ideas from Stoicism that have had a profound effect on my life. My goal is to convince you to give them a try.

Now, it might have become clear at this point that I am not an academic philosophy scholar. But, my knowledge of Stoicism has come from real-world application of the ideas. This book is not supposed to be an academic analysis of the ancient ideas. I'd like to think of it as more of a call to action.

I've done my absolute best to represent the Stoics' ideas as clearly as possible. Any errors are mine rather than the Stoics' – so please forgive me (I'm only human). When you're talking about philosophy there are many nuances and areas that scholars spend a lot of time fiercely debating. I'm not in the game for that so if I unintentionally misrepresent your favourite Stoic idea, be a Stoic and forgive me. Thanks in advance.

PUTTING STOICISM INTO PRACTICE

As soon as I'd finished writing my first book, I didn't realize how quickly the ideas and philosophy in it would be put to use. At the start of 2020, we were all hit with the global coronavirus pandemic.

The early days of the pandemic were scary and the fear of the unknown made things worse. We didn't fully understand the virus and we weren't sure what would happen. At the beginning of the first lockdown, fear levels were at an all-time-high. At one point, it felt like the world had gone crazy as people battled over toilet roll. The only thing that made the absurdity of the situation any better – although only slightly – was the vast number of high-quality memes flying around on the Internet. (Ah, memes … the world can be on fire and in utter chaos and there will always be someone out there trying to make us laugh. This is something I love and admire about the human spirit.)

During this time I leant heavily into Stoic philosophy. It helped me immensely when it felt like the apocalypse was taking place. It also allowed me to find objectivity in what was happening around me and encouraged me to put my attention in the right place. I spent a lot of time digging deep into the philosophy and this brought me a huge amount of comfort.

My first book, *How to be Comfortable with Being Uncomfortable*, was released in the middle of the first lockdown in the UK.

Amazingly, despite closed warehouses, furlough and no book-stores being open, it made it out into the world. It was born into chaos but this seemed appropriate for a book that focused on mental resilience.

The response to the book was lovely. So many readers reached out to share their stories with me and to ask questions. It seemed like the right time for the book to come out and I was so pleased that we managed to release it during lockdown, despite the various hurdles.

Around the time of the book launch, I found myself creating various lockdown challenges inspired by the Stoics' ideas on control. We will visit this concept in more detail later, but the Stoics encouraged us to focus on our response to external events. In doing this, we regain our power in a situation. There were so many restrictions in place during lockdown but this didn't mean that I couldn't continue to challenge myself … I could focus on how I responded to these restrictions and choose to make the best out of a difficult situation.

Rather than let the lockdown limit me, I decided to still go on adventures – but at home. I love climbing and mountaineering but couldn't get to the mountains, so I decided that I would bring the mountains to me … and set out to climb Mount Everest on my staircase. Yes, this was a totally ridiculous experience.

Everest is 8,848 metres in height and, after some maths and measuring, I calculated that I needed to climb and descend my stairs 2,137 times to cover that distance. Unsurprisingly, the experience lasted a while … I kept a solid pace throughout, but it took me 21 hours to complete the climb. I did this over 8 days and ended up burning a lot of calories. It was the weirdest mountaineering experience I've ever had.

One of the highlights of my climb was the interactions and exchanges on social media. The sense of community was brilliant and I managed to recruit some "virtual climbing partners". I was even offered Sherpa support from an Everest expedition company!

A few weeks later, I continued in the spirit of lockdown challenges and ran a marathon in my garden. After whipping out the calculator, I discovered that it would take 4,802 lengths of the garden to cover the distance of a marathon. It was another utterly ridiculous experience.

I completed the marathon but it took a lot longer than I thought it would (I had to keep stopping and starting due to the short length of the garden). My neighbours probably thought I was crazy. Their children did make signs for me, though, and hung them over the fence to support me, which was very kind.

Lots of people tell me how absurd these two events sound – but I completely disagree. These experiences are some of the most memorable things I've ever done. It's all about how you view the situation. When I look back on the first time we went into a lockdown in the UK, I now have special memories. It taught me so much about making the best out of a tough situation.

Granted, these examples aren't things the Stoics were directly doing. But it's what studying their ideas inspired me to do. You just never know what direction these ideas will take you in – hopefully further than the top of your stairs!

THE ANTI-BUCKET LIST

An idea that I mentioned in my first book was the "anti-bucket list" and lots of people connected to the concept. When I've been out and about talking on podcasts or doing interviews, this is an idea that I enjoy talking about. It's directly inspired by the Stoics and, as you will see later, it's something that I would love to contribute to the philosophy. But I'm getting carried away ... First things first.

The anti-bucket list is the opposite of a bucket list. So maybe let's start with that. A bucket list is essentially a list of things you want to do before you die; before you "kick the bucket" as they say. Things like seeing the Northern Lights, writing a book, going to Las Vegas or learning a language might be on the list. It will be different for everyone. The anti-bucket list is the opposite – it's what you want to avoid doing in your life at all costs, things that terrify you and make you uncomfortable. Examples could be giving blood, holding a spider or swimming in deep water. Like the bucket list, the anti-bucket list will also be unique to each and every one of us.

As adults, it's easy to avoid doing things that scare us and make us uncomfortable. We can choose to completely avoid something. For example, you might have a real problem with dogs, dentists or heights and deliberately avoid these situations, limiting your life. The thing is, whoever you are, it's difficult to completely escape all fear. We are human beings and fear is an emotion that we will all experience. It's normal. We need to accept this and learn to work with it.

The idea of the anti-bucket list is to turn this fear into play – two words that you don't normally associate with each other! Facing our fears is an incredible way to grow as human beings. It's also a brilliantly Stoic thing to do.

My anti-bucket list was very long when I was at the peak of my anxiety. Trivial things were on the list that most people wouldn't even consider – simple daily activities like catching the bus or driving on the motorway were overwhelming for me. Over time, I would tick things off the list by actively seeking them out. This helped so much with my confidence. Slowly I pushed myself further. I had a fear of needles so went and got acupuncture (that first session was intense). I also started picking up house spiders. OK – I started picking up *small* house spiders. These challenges had a huge impact on my life and I noticed a significant shift in my mindset. I'm not exactly fearless now, and I still have plenty of things on my anti-bucket list, but working through them has been empowering.

There's a psychological technique in use today called "fear exposure" that therapists use to help patients deal with phobias. By exposing them to the things that they are afraid of, they become desensitized to them over time. The anti-bucket list works in a similar way – scary things that would be easy to avoid become opportunities to grow. We revisit this idea later in the book – but start thinking now about what would go on your list.

Like the lockdown challenges, the anti-bucket list has grown out of having a foundational understanding of Stoic philosophy. This is the beauty of exposing ourselves to new ways of looking at things – it can act as a stepping stone to other viewpoints. I'm confident that after reading about the Stoics, you will be able to extract the elements that are relevant to you and incorporate them into your life. I'm excited for you.

So, that's how I got into Stoic philosophy and how I've been testing myself with these ancient ideas. I've learned so much in the process and will continue to use Stoicism as a tool to support and develop myself. Anyway, I'm going to let the philosophy do the talking now.

HOW TO USE THIS BOOK

This isn't just a book for reading; it's a book for doing. In essence, there are a couple of things that this book aims to do:

1. Give you a clear understanding of what Stoicism is
2. Share a bunch of practical exercises to test it out

I've broken the book down into three main parts. The first part – "Ben's Guide to Stoicism" – is an introduction to the core ideas of the Stoics and explores a little of their history. Don't worry, this isn't a dry academic textbook, it's just setting you up with the basics so that you have context for everything.

The second part of the book is the juicy bit. "The Stoic Principles" is where I give my top 10 game-changing ideas from Stoicism. There are exercises, challenges and lots of stuff for you to have fun with here.

The final part – "Putting Stoicism into Practice" – explores some interesting ways to bring these Stoic ideas together in challenges of differing length and complexity. There are also resources that might be helpful for you on your Stoic journey.

When using this book, I think the most important thing is to actually test out these Stoic ideas in the real world. Use them when out and about. Play around with them and see what works for you. Tackle the challenges head-on and embrace any discomfort along the way with a positive mindset.

Epictetus, one of the most famous Stoics of all time, has a great quote about the importance of actually getting out there and putting these ideas to the test:

"We might be fluent in the classroom but drag us out into practice and we're miserably shipwrecked."

Epictetus

So, don't let that be you. Don't just read about all of this and not put it into practice – it won't have the same impact. Epictetus wouldn't be happy with you.

The Stoics had a word they used for all of this – *askêsis*. It essentially means "training". Like getting out there and walking the walk. Not just talking the talk. This was an incredibly important part of the philosophy. Action is something that makes Stoicism what it is. Without it, the philosophy is just a bunch of words.

Along with action, I also recommend reflection and note-taking as a way to engage further with these ideas. Grab a notepad, journal or diary and use this to write about what you discover in these pages. The Stoics were huge fans of the journal and, as we go through the book, you will be encouraged to test out journaling activities with each principle. These aren't particularly time consuming and will prompt you to think about how these ideas are relevant to you. Or you could take notes on your phone – you have no excuses.

I really hope that the ideas that follow will bring insight and knowledge into your life. The Stoics were truly great thinkers and have some wonderful ideas for facing the chaos of life.

PART 1

BEN'S GUIDE TO STOICISM

Welcome to my guide to Stoicism. This section of the book is an overview of the philosophy and will give you a basic understanding of what Stoicism is and where it came from. It will set you up perfectly for the main chunk of the book – the 10 game-changing principles and the practical bits that follow.

Think of this as a mini-introduction to the philosophy. It's not super-duper detailed, but will provide a solid grounding in these ideas and a base for taking everything further as you progress through these pages. A quick note – I have included a Stoic Cheat Sheet at the end of the book that summarizes the key themes and terms I mention. This is a great place to visit to recap any of the technical content.

1

WHAT'S ALL THIS STOICISM BUSINESS, ANYWAY?

So, let's start at the beginning: what is Stoicism?

Stoicism is an ancient Greek philosophy that has one main purpose – to help people live better lives. The philosophy has lots of great ideas within it but its number one goal is for us to learn how to live "the good life". Ultimately, to flourish as human beings. To be happy. To be able to handle what comes our way. To be ready to surf the wave of life.

The Stoics had a word they would use for this mindset – *eudaimonia*. No, it's not a new genre of European Techno music, it's a word that essentially means happiness. Sort of. It's hard to translate – maybe think of it as something similar to equanimity. Finding balance. Cultivating wellbeing. Being able to spin the plates and keep things ticking along despite the challenges that life throws at us. *Eudaimonia* can be seen as the foundation of the philosophy. Everything that you read about can be traced back to this idea. All roads lead to happiness/ balance/tranquillity (in a way).

The Stoics have many suggestions on how to achieve this mindset and live a better life. However, they mainly encourage us to do this by cultivating a good and virtuous character. That may sound a bit lofty and grand but the idea of "virtue" is integral to Stoicism. The Stoics believed that your character was everything and the most important aspect of who you are. To live virtuously means to live by an ethical code that the Stoics

3

spent time thinking about. Ethics were extremely important to them. This is a big part of the philosophy and how we conduct ourselves is a reflection of how philosophical we are. Whatever challenges we face in life, there is a philosophical way to deal with things and an unphilosophical way to deal with them – the moral high ground or the low path through questionable morality. Helping a frail elder across the road or stealing their groceries while laughing like a maniac.

Developing a virtuous character sounds pretty intense but it's essentially a process of self-reflection. The Stoics looked at how they were living their lives and asked themselves if they were being the best version of themselves in that moment. As for a lot of things in Stoicism, this concept also has a name: *aretê*. It essentially means being the best possible version of yourself in every instance. Of course, that's impossible and things will go wrong (we're only human, after all) but the point is that this is an ongoing process and we should keep trying to be the best we can possibly be. It's basically good judgement – just be a decent person (and try to be a decent person all the time).

The Stoics believed that if you can build a good character, you can become happy and balanced. Or, if you're being fancy, if you live a life of virtue and *aretê*, you can achieve *eudaimonia*.

I like the fact that Stoicism puts the responsibility for happiness into our hands. We can create our own happiness – it's not dependent on external things. We are responsible for this. No one else. This personal responsibility has similarities to Buddhism. In Buddhism, happiness comes from within and the Stoics believed the same thing. It's internal. Not external. It's not about Lamborghinis and auto-flushing gold toilets; it's about how you feel inside. It's all about your perception of the world.

So, how do we build a good character? And what exactly is living a virtuous existence? Well, the Stoics were guided by something called "The Cardinal Virtues". These are regarded as the benchmark for becoming a "good" human being.

THE CARDINAL VIRTUES

Now, the Stoics didn't just pluck these virtues out of thin air. Plato, the Greek philosopher, established them and the Stoics thought they were spot on. They decided to live with these ideas at the forefront of their minds and make them a fundamental part of their philosophy.

When the Stoics talk about "virtues", there are four that they consider to be the most important. These are the qualities of character that the Stoics believed we should strive to bring into our lives. They are:

1. Wisdom
2. Justice
3. Fortitude
4. Temperance

WISDOM

Wisdom (sometimes referred to as "Prudence" by the Stoics) is the ability to understand the world around us and make sound decisions in life based on this understanding. It's also the ability to know what we can and can't control in life (we'll talk more on this later).

Stoic wisdom is:

1. The ability to make wise and sensible decisions.
2. Knowing that complaining about the weather isn't going to change it.
3. Understanding that the best course of action for a lot of problems we face in life can be found within philosophy.

According to the Stoics, attaining "wisdom" will allow us to handle whatever life throws at us. The Stoics believed that philosophy was the greatest source of this wisdom so therefore it made sense to invest time in studying it. This was certainly true for me – when I was in a particularly dark place in my life, I found philosophy incredibly helpful. (Philosophy actually means "a love of wisdom", so it ties in with this cardinal virtue.)

JUSTICE

Justice as a virtue is essentially being a fair and decent human being. Pretty straightforward, right? It's the ability to be kind to others, irrespective of how annoying they are. It's also synonymous with our personal responsibility to work toward a better humanity. Justice is:

1. When someone is rude to us, we don't freak out and start shouting at the top of our voices at them.
2. We are kind to people and fair in how we deal with them.
3. We aspire to make the world a better place for our existence.

This is all about equality and fairness – something as relevant in today's world as it was 2,000 years ago. The Stoics spoke about how, although we are individuals, we are part of humanity at large and that our actions have an impact on everyone, but I'll come back to that in the principles section.

FORTITUDE

Fortitude is the ability to endure hardships and handle adversity effectively. It's the strength of character that allows us to face our fears, deal with life's curveballs and live courageously. In fact, sometimes the word "courage" is used instead of fortitude for this virtue. The word "resilience" also fits perfectly here. Fortitude can be seen as:

1. The ability to handle setbacks and rise up to the challenges in front of us.

2. Dealing with discomfort gracefully (without complaining every five seconds).
3. The courage to stand up for what we believe in even if that will be difficult to do.

This is a virtue exemplified by grit, endurance and resilience. I'll often think about someone battling arctic conditions on some epic polar trek when I think about this virtue. In reality, it doesn't have to be that extreme – you don't have to travel to one of the poles to experience it. Simply enduring a long queue, handling discomfort or stepping outside of our comfort zones can be just as effective.

TEMPERANCE

Temperance is essentially self-control. It could also be interpreted as discipline and the ability to stick with difficult things and situations. This one is quite self-explanatory. Temperance is:

1. Being able to say no.
2. Being able to cultivate discipline and commit to our goals.
3. Being able to *not* order pizza for the third day in a row.

This virtue is intertwined with our emotions and how we manage them. Think of it as the ability to stay in control of our minds, irrespective of what happens to us. We'll be looking at managing strong emotions later in the book, so your temperance will be put into practice at that point.

The thing about The Cardinal Virtues is that they come from Greek words that are a little tricky to translate. They aren't straightforward conversions and some of the subtleties can get lost in translation. This is an area that scholars often debate over but as long as you get the gist of the virtues in this section, I'm happy.

The Stoics believe that by using these virtues as guiding ethical principles, we will achieve *eudaimonia* (happiness/tranquillity/balance/flourishing/wellbeing). These are the characteristics that make you a good person, and they will help you to live a better life. I'd suggest trying to hold them in your mind as you work through this book. Think about how the Stoics felt it was important to have a decent character. And refer as often as you can to these four cardinal virtues for guidance.

MY STOIC LION

Before we move on, I want to share with you a quick way to easily remember The Cardinal Virtues.

Picture a lion reading a book while taking a sip of water. Now picture the lion getting up, putting on a judge's wig and entering a court room. Have you got that image in your mind? OK great! It's a little bizarre, I know. But strange and powerful images can be wonderful mnemonic devices (quick tricks to memorize stuff).

The lion represents the *fortitude* virtue. That's easy to remember – lions are strong, brave and fearless animals. The book represents *wisdom* – that's also pretty obvious as books are the ultimate source of wisdom. The water is a little more abstract but will hopefully make sense. It represents *temperance* – imagine that the Lion has cut out all caffeine and now only drinks water. Nothing else. This lion is unbelievably self-disciplined with what it puts into its body. Thus, the water representing self-control or temperance. Are you still with me? Finally, the judge's wig and courtroom represent *justice* – but you probably guessed that one.

This might seem a little abstract, but when you first come across the four virtues, it's easy to forget them. Using a simple trick like this can help to keep them in your mind until you don't have to use the mnemonic anymore. It's quick and effective but feel free to alter this if you're not comfortable with wig-wearing, self-disciplined lions.

HOW TO CONTROL THE UNCONTROLLABLE

The Stoics' take on control is something that has truly helped me in life – so much so, that I based the name of this book on it.

The Stoics believed that we have little control over external events (basically, much of the stuff that happens to us). Life is uncertain and we can't control outcomes. However, they did believe that we could control our response to those external events. So, by focusing on our reaction to the uncontrollable, we bring some semblance of control into the equation.

So, can we *actually* control the uncontrollable? If so, how?

Well, we can't *directly* control the uncontrollable. Think about the weather – we can't make it rain (even if we do a rain dance and shake a stick at the sky). We also can't make the rain stop (as much as we might will it to) ... However, we can use an umbrella. And we can water our plants with a hosepipe when there is no rain. We can *respond* to the uncontrollable by taking action. It's about what we choose to do when facing events outside of our control.

With the title of this book, I'm not saying we can actually control uncontrollable events. But ... we can control what we do next. This is how we control the uncontrollable. It's essentially a management strategy. It's about remembering our umbrellas, responding to the chaos of life with a rational approach, and bringing solutions to problems by focusing on the next steps.

I'll pass the baton on to the Stoic philosopher Epictetus – he states it succinctly:

"It's not what happens to you, but how you react to it that matters."

Epictetus

By choosing to focus on our response to what happens to us, we bring power back into our hands. That awful thing might have taken place, but we can pick where we go from here and how we deal with it. This is very much a mindset thing. And it's a wonderful way to deal with setbacks and hardships.

This theme weaves its way through the philosophy and is such a huge part of Stoicism. In my first book, I referred to this concept as Stoicism's "Golden Rule". And I'm going to stand by this. It's how I visualize this idea in my mind. You'll encounter "The Stoic Golden Rule" throughout this book, but if we're being technical about it, there is actually another name for this idea – "The Dichotomy of Control". This expression wasn't used by the ancients and is relatively new. But it's frequently used by Modern Stoics so it's worth knowing.

The reason it's called The Dichotomy of Control is because there are two components of control. We have a clear split – things that we can do something about (our response) and things that we can't (pretty much everything else). Knowing the difference is important for a Stoic.

Zeno, the founder of Stoicism, had a great metaphor for all of this. Imagine a dog tied to the back of a cart with a leash. The dog can't control where the cart goes so has two options … It can either choose to go in the direction the cart takes it and trot along behind it, or the dog can resist, in which case, it will get dragged.

The dog represents us and the cart represents life. We have a choice – to go with the flow – or be dragged through life (potentially kicking and screaming). Yes, we have some flexibility (like the dog has with the leash), but the cart of life will keep on rolling … So, we better keep up!

By understanding what we can and can't control, we can stop wasting time worrying about things that we can't change or do anything about. This is very helpful. We can then focus our attention in the right place.

INDIFFERENCES

The Stoics believed that we should be *indifferent* toward the things that are outside of our control. This is an interesting concept in the philosophy.

What does it mean to be *indifferent*? Well, it means that we don't weight things outside of our control too heavily. And that we certainly wouldn't use them as a way to judge others. For example, the Stoics thought that all of the following were *indifferences*: money, health, reputation, possessions and beauty.

These things are all pretty much outside of our control. Yes, we can do things to help influence them. We can eat well to optimize our health, but, as we all know, this doesn't stop some random illness or problem cropping up. The same is true for money – we can work hard but someone might rob us, or inflation can cause our wealth to decrease in value or we might make a bad investment. The list goes on.

The Stoics claimed that these *indifferences* don't intrinsically make you a better person. You can be extremely wealthy and be an awful person. You can also be extremely wealthy and be a really kind and caring person. Money is a variable. People with less money can be decent or horrible. It's about how they live their life – is their character good? This is what the Stoics valued.

They would say the same for health. You can be sick, but this doesn't have to destroy your character. You can be terribly ill, but still be a nice person. Again, for beauty – the way you look doesn't make you a good or bad person, and our possessions don't define who we are. They can easily break or be taken from us. The important thing to the Stoics was your character.

The reality is, most of us would rather be healthy than sick, and have enough money to survive. This is perfectly normal and a very acceptable desire from all of us. The Stoics acknowledged this and called these preferences *"preferred indifferences"*.

However, they are still seen as *indifferences* and ultimately something that we shouldn't weight as overly important.

THE STOIC ARCHER

The Stoics believed that a lot of dissatisfaction in life comes from having unrealistic expectations of reality. If we think that we have more control over life than we actually do, we get frustrated and disappointed when things don't go to plan. They have a great solution for managing this – they encourage us to remember that nothing is guaranteed. There are so many variables at play in life that things will go wrong. Not always, but life is unpredictable, so we should expect the unexpected. There will be big and small blips in our plans.

To help us build this idea into our mindsets, the Stoics have a concept called "The Reserve Clause" – originally known as *hupexairesis*. This is pretty much the equivalent of adding the expression "fate permitting" to the end of our sentences when discussing plans. For example: "I will go to the beach tomorrow, fate permitting". Or "I will have takeaway for dinner, fate permitting".

We don't have to say this out loud all the time for everything that we do, but we can use it as a mental reminder that nothing is guaranteed. I can intend to go to the beach tomorrow, but it might rain. My car might break down. A bunch of wild badgers might start attacking me. Well, I'm pretty confident that the last one won't happen but you get the idea. Things can get in the way of my intention. To think otherwise is being deluded. It's important for us to remember this. It doesn't mean that we shouldn't ever plan or expect things, it just means that we need to be aware that there is a lot of stuff that is beyond our control.

The Stoics have an example called "The Stoic Archer". Imagine an archer: they raise their bow and aim it at the target.

They intend to hit the bullseye but as soon as they release the arrow, they have no control over what happens. There might be a gust of wind that blows the arrow off course. The target might move. Some more wild badgers might get in the way (again). There are lots of things that could mean the outcome doesn't mirror the intention.

Not expecting or feeling entitled to an outcome is the Stoic way of avoiding disappointment – it's about doing the best we can in any given situation and accepting that the result might not always be what we want. But we can handle whatever happens because we can choose how we respond to it.

THE STRUCTURE OF STOIC PHILOSOPHY

When I first got into Stoicism, I wasn't aware of the structure that I'm about to share with you. I just dove straight in and started reading as much as I could. Over time I learned how the philosophy was divided up. When you read the Stoics, this isn't glaringly obvious at first, so it's useful to be aware of this.

In Stoic philosophy there are three main areas that the Stoics would teach to their students: Logic, Ethics and Physics. These are slightly different to how we perceive them today.

LOGIC

Logic is mainly about applying reasoning to the way we think. It's actually similar to modern psychology as it focuses on our judgements and perceptions. The Stoics took this idea and turned it into a "discipline". They called this the "Discipline of Assent". It sounds fancy, but this is essentially the application of Logic and reasoning to the way we live our lives. It's the ability to stay in control when facing tough emotions and make informed judgements – very practical indeed!

ETHICS

Ethics is pretty much as it sounds. It looks at how we behave and what is considered good, bad or indifferent. This gets referred to as the "Discipline of Action" and predominantly focuses on our behaviour but also looks at our relationship with the rest of humanity. So, maybe now is a good time to brush up on your table manners ...

PHYSICS

Physics is about the big picture – the cosmic order of things. Overall, it is philosophy and a touch of theology. As a discipline, this gets called the "Discipline of Desire". Interestingly, this discipline looks at what we can and can't control in life (The Stoic Golden Rule) and encourages us to think about the cosmic order of things. It also looks at what we desire – but I guess that might have been obvious, given the name. It's worth noting that this discipline is *not* based on calculating scientific forces like a modern physicist would do.

These three themes and disciplines are worth being aware of as they crop up all the time in Stoicism. Lots of Modern Stoic philosophers and scholars will approach things from these angles but they do all melt into each other though, so I won't be dividing up the content in this book according to this philosophical structure.

THE STOIC GODS

It's helpful to know that the ancient Stoics' theological world view was pantheistic – this is essentially the idea that God *is* the universe. And we are part of that universe. If you read the Stoics, you will often find Zeus cropping up, especially if you read Epictetus. The thing is, the Stoics didn't think of Zeus as a major bloke (the king of the gods) in the sky who hung around in the clouds smoking a mystical pipe ... Zeus *was* the universe. Zeus was synonymous with nature and represented *everything* in the universe.

In Stoic philosophy there was also the mention of other gods (not just Zeus). The gods, in a way, were representations of forces. One of the most famous being Fortuna – she was a god that essentially anthropomorphized fate. It's worth knowing that any of the other gods mentioned by the Stoics were pretty much different aspects or manifestations of Zeus. All roads lead to Zeus ... How about that for a slogan?!

If you are an atheist or closely follow a religion, the idea of believing in Zeus can be a deal-breaker. However, in Modern Stoicism, Zeus and the other gods aren't really a feature. In fact, modern scholars don't write about the gods in the same way as the ancients did. Modern Stoicism doesn't focus on this aspect of the philosophy and can easily function without it.

I think it's important to be aware of all of this, though, because if you read the ancient Stoics, which I highly recommend, you will encounter the gods. This brief overview will help it to make sense in a modern context and help you to not fixate on the use of the word "gods".

It's worth remembering at this point that Stoicism is a philosophy rather than a religion. Although the ancients mentioned the gods, the Stoic ideas don't require us to worship Zeus which is great for two reasons. If you already have a religion in your life, Stoic philosophy can work beautifully in partnership with it; incorporating these concepts into your life won't require you to abandon your faith. If you are an atheist or agnostic, Stoicism will also work beautifully with your world view – these ideas are predominately based on reason and logic and complement modern scientific thought well. You do not need to believe in God and/or gods to be a Stoic.

So, whatever your cosmological, theological or philosophical background, Stoicism has got you covered!

THE STOIC MISCONCEPTION

Before we go any further, it's important to mention something super-important. Stoicism often gets confused with the word stoic. Confused? I don't blame you! Stoicism with a capital "S" refers to the ancient Greek philosophy. Yes, what this book is all about. Whereas "stoic" with a lowercase "s" can be used to express when someone is "unemotional" or "represses their emotions", a "just get on with it" attitude.

It's a common misconception. Maybe THE main misconception about Stoicism. Being a Stoic doesn't mean that you are a cold and emotionless statue that doesn't cry at Disney movies. Stoicism *isn't* about repressing emotions. It talks of not letting emotions control you, but that's different to repression and we'll explore this later on in the book.

Basically, just know that Stoicism doesn't make you a cold emotionless robot. None of the Stoics were like this and it's important to remember that.

So now you know what Stoicism is (and what it's not), I'm going to put my history cap on and summarize thousands of years of Stoic history in a few pages ...

2

A BRIEF HISTORY OF STOICISM

In my eyes there are three important influences in Stoicism's history. The Greeks who began Stoicism, the Roman Stoics who followed (which includes most of the Stoic names you'll have heard of) and the Modern Stoics. All have shaped the philosophy and contributed to its development. Let's start at the beginning.

THE GREEK BIT

In approximately 300 BCE, a man called Zeno founded Stoicism. Zeno was from a place in Cyprus called Citium. Thus, he was officially known as Zeno of Citium.

There's an interesting story about how he came to start the first school of Stoic philosophy. Zeno was travelling by boat and was shipwrecked. He survived but lost all of his cargo (an absolute fortune). This event proved to be a real catalyst for change in his life. After the shipwreck he found himself in Athens where he developed an interest in philosophy. At the time, Athens was *the* place to be if you wanted to learn about philosophy.

One day, Zeno found himself in a bookstore reading about Socrates. (A quick side note here: Socrates (470-399 BCE) was the "Grandfather of Western Philosophy". Often, he is credited as the most important philosopher of all time. He extensively relied on logic and reasoning in his dialogues and this heavily influenced the Stoics.) As Zeno was thumbing through the book, he asked the shop owner where he could find someone like Socrates – a philosopher. As it happened – or so the legend goes – a philosopher called Crates of Thebes was walking by at that very moment. I know, really convenient, right? Zeno decided to start an apprenticeship with Crates and began studying philosophy with him.

Crates was from a philosophical school called the Cynics. They were quite extreme; think of them as hardcore monks. I remember hearing someone describe the Cynics as the "trolls of Ancient Greece" and I quite like this description. They would walk backwards in public and deliberately trudge through crowds coming out of theatres. They loved doing difficult and provocative things. As we explore Stoicism, you will see how the Cynics have influenced them with this particular concept.

There's a great story about Crates making Zeno carry a giant bowl of soup across Athens as part of his philosophical training. Zeno was embarrassed about having to do this as carrying soup supposedly had a stigma around it – only poor people would do this – and as Zeno felt self-conscious, Crates decided to teach Zeno a lesson. While they were walking, Crates smashed the bowl of soup and covered Zeno in it. Crates told Zeno to get a grip and stop worrying about what everyone was thinking about him! Those weren't his exact words but you get the sentiment.

After studying with Crates for some time, Zeno went on to explore philosophy from other schools. Eventually he decided to take the leap into the unknown and set up his own school of philosophy. This was a combination of the ideas he had already encountered and his own. Stoicism was born.

Zeno started lecturing about his ideas under a giant porch in Athens called the *Stoa Poikile*. The porch/building was covered in fine paintings that depicted military battles and mythical stories. The direct translation of the word for the building means "painted porch" and you can see how the word "Stoicism" has come from this. The *Stoa Poikile* was where you went to learn about Stoicism. Simple!

It's interesting that the Stoics named their philosophy after a geographic location, rather than Zeno the founder. Lots of philosophies and religions are named after the person who created them but the Stoics believed that no one was perfect, so opted for a location, rather than a person.

Zeno's lectures were open for anyone to join and he developed quite a following. People came from all over to listen to him talk about philosophy. It was street philosophy, for the people, at its finest.

Eventually it came time for Zeno to step down from his role and appoint the next head of the Stoic school. He chose a man named Cleanthes.

Cleanthes was a diligent student of Stoicism and had attended Zeno's lectures for many years before taking over from him. The story is that Cleanthes came to Athens to better himself and eventually ended up running a school of philosophy. So it seems like he achieved his original goal.

When Cleanthes first arrived in Athens, he had empty pockets but a serious work ethic. He was a reputable boxer and had a very physical job – he was a water carrier and would transport water all over Athens. This financially supported his philosophical study and became a way for him to test out Stoicism in the real world – through arduous conditions.

Cleanthes was famed for his slow and steady approach to learning. People would refer to him as "the donkey" in a rather derogatory way, but Cleanthes thought that the comparison wasn't so bad – a donkey was hardworking and able to carry heavy loads. He felt that this meant he would be able to carry Stoicism on his back as he led the Stoic school.

Cleanthes wrote multiple books but as with most of the writing from this period of time, they have been lost to history. He was exactly 100 when he passed away.

After Cleanthes, we have Chrysippus. He was the third head of the Stoic school and helped to progress Stoic thought further. He had a love of running which seemed to influence his approach to Stoic philosophy. The competitiveness and discipline translated directly into his attitude. Chrysippus wanted Stoicism to win.

He studied other rival philosophical schools so that he could develop arguments and counter-arguments. This helped him to push Stoic ideas by looking for weaknesses in them, and then improving them. He was intellectual, sharp and quick. He was also an incredibly prolific writer. Apparently, he wrote over 705 books – a serious body of work.

Chrysippus was also a bit of a rock star – he was the first Stoic to start lecturing outside of the *Stoa Poikile* and taught philosophy on larger stages in a variety of different venues. He really put Stoicism on the map. So much so that his face was stuck on coins after his death.

Chrysippus had a rather unusual end to his life. The legend goes that he actually died of laughter. He was having lunch one day and spotted a donkey chewing on a nearby hedge. Chrysippus said something along the lines of, "Would you like some wine with that?" and thought that his own joke was so funny that he died laughing. This story goes against the image of Stoics being emotionless and cold. It's totally ridiculous and makes me think of the Monty Python sketch where someone invents the funniest joke in the world and uses it during the war as a secret weapon.

The heads of Stoicism continued to change as the philosophy prospered in Ancient Greece. Unfortunately, most of the literature and books written during this period have been lost. And yes, that includes Chrysippus' epic collection of over 705 books.

We know what we know about the Greek part of Stoicism thanks to various people writing *about* the Stoics. Thankfully, not all of the ancient Stoics' actual work has been lost – as you're about to find out. Eventually the philosophy made its way to Rome, a place where people were better at not losing books!

THE ROMAN BIT

While the books from the Greek part of Stoic history have been lost, the Roman bit has plenty of surviving material. This was a prolific time for Stoic literature and there is some great content for us to sink our teeth into. In fact, most of the quotes in this book come from this era. You can think of it as the golden age of Stoicism.

Rather than a chronological, historical line through this period of time, I'm going to give you a brief biography of the most important Stoic philosophers from the Roman bit to give you a sense of the era. Plus, you will be encountering these Stoics throughout the book, so you really should get to know them.

There are four Stoic philosophers from Ancient Rome to have on your radar – Seneca, Musonius Rufus, Epictetus and Marcus Aurelius. Let me introduce them to you:

LUCIUS ANNAEUS SENECA (4 BCE–65 CE)

Seneca was a Roman Stoic philosopher and contributed greatly to the progression of Stoicism. He was born in Spain but raised in Rome where he studied philosophy. He became a statesman, writer and eventually an advisor to the Emperor Nero. This ended badly when Nero ordered Seneca to kill himself. Nero accused Seneca of being part of an assassination plot against him. It is likely that this accusation was false. But Seneca calmly took his life and accepted his fate without complaint.

In my first book I described Seneca as a Roman "Oprah". I'd like to stick with that here. I feel that Seneca was one of the greatest self-help gurus of the Roman era. I say this because a lot of his work comes in the form of letters to friends and family. These letters offered advice on a wide range of topics from dealing with setbacks to living with purpose. Even today these letters are incredibly relevant as they are packed with practical wisdom that has stood the test of time.

Seneca also wrote plays, essays and a satire. All of this content has helped us to gain a deeper understanding of Stoic philosophy. I highly recommend spending some time reading through his works.

A side note – there is a reading list that you can work through at the end of the book called How to Build a Stoic Library. This lists all of the books I mention in these pages.

MUSONIUS RUFUS (20/30–101 CE)
Born in Italy, Rufus was considered to be the "Roman Socrates", exemplifying self-discipline and living a virtuous life. He became famous for teaching philosophy and had a huge impact on spreading Stoic thought. He was very much someone who embraced discomfort and would see it as part and parcel of life.

He also believed in equality and wrote passionately about women's rights to study philosophy and be treated as equals. This would have been considered incredibly progressive at the time. But Stoic philosophy focused on virtue and this transcended many of the limits and injustices of the age. We know that Rufus was a fan of simplicity in living – basic food, clothing and furnishings being his preference. This humble attitude can be seen in the snippets of his writing that remain.

Rufus was exiled multiple times throughout his life due to different Emperors having different rules for different philosophers. He frequently found himself in challenging environments but leant into his Stoic philosophy to endure these hard times.

When he was not being sent off to faraway places in exile, he was a well-known Stoic teacher. Epictetus was his most famous student and went on to greatly impact the philosophy. So, I think it's fair to say that he did a pretty good job of passing on these ideas.

EPICTETUS (55–135 CE)

Epictetus was born in what we now call Turkey. He was the son of a slave and born into slavery. Epictetus means "acquired one" in Greek – a reminder of how the first part of his life was lived.

Epictetus was lame and walked with a limp – one theory was that his master twisted his leg until it snapped as a form of punishment. We can't be sure of this but it was certainly during his years as a slave that the injury occurred. Epictetus gained his freedom at the age of 30 as the law at the time meant that slaves became free after hitting that milestone in their lives. Upon gaining his freedom, he went on to study philosophy which is where he met Rufus. Eventually, Epictetus set up his own school of Stoicism.

Interestingly, he never wrote anything down. Thankfully, his student Arrian did. This is how we know about Epictetus' take on Stoicism. Every book or work that has Epictetus' name on it was technically written by Arrian.

You'll notice that there is a heavy emphasis in Epictetus' writings on how we respond to things outside of our control. Given that he was born into slavery and had to face particularly challenging circumstances at the start of his life, it makes total sense that The Stoic Golden Rule was so important to him.

He has a collection of essays that are very popular but his handbook for living (*The Enchiridion*) is a great way to learn about his take on Stoicism. It's a quick read and a wonderful introduction to his thinking.

MARCUS AURELIUS (121–180 CE)

Marcus Aurelius is probably the most famous Stoic philosopher to have ever walked the Earth. He was the Roman Emperor from 161–180 CE and arguably the most powerful human being on the planet at the time. During his reign, he had to deal with wars, treason, the death of his children and many more challenging situations.

Aurelius also had to face a devastating pandemic called the "Antonine Plague" (the plague was actually named after him – Marcus Aurelius Antoninus). This was one of the worst plagues in European history, killing 5 million people. It might have even killed Aurelius himself. Handling this situation and managing an entire Empire during this time would have been incredibly demanding.

This is where philosophy comes into the equation. Stoicism acted as his guide and helped him to manage his responses to all of these setbacks and challenges. It was during this incredibly difficult period that he wrote his *Meditations*. Out of desperate and demanding times, he created one of the most influential pieces of philosophical works in history.

Meditations was never meant for publication. It was actually his diary or journal. This was essentially a way for him to reflect on Stoic philosophy and ensure that he was living in alignment with these ideas. It's the only writing we have from Aurelius, but it's absolutely packed with practical wisdom and is truly timeless.

Aurelius was a popular Emperor and well loved by the Romans. His ability to stay true to the Stoic path, especially when it would have been so easy for him to be corrupted, is testament to the power of the philosophy. And it's also testament to his commitment to these ideas.

THE BEST OF THE REST

There are many more Stoics to discover from the Roman bit, but these four, in my opinion, have had the greatest impact on the philosophy. I'm therefore not going to overwhelm you with bits and bobs from the not-so-famous Roman Stoics as I think it's important to become familiar with these guys first. I will mention other Stoics throughout the book, but the vast majority of what you encounter will come from Seneca, Rufus, Epictetus and Aurelius.

If you're keen to expand your knowledge of the actual Stoics and want to dive into the history of both the Greek and Roman bits in more detail, I have several book recommendations for this later on.

THE MODERN BIT

After the Romans, there weren't many movers and shakers in Stoicism for quite some time. Christianity took over and led the way for hundreds of years while Stoicism sat patiently on the sidelines. At one point, there was nearly a comeback when Justus Lipsius (1547–1606) tried to merge Christianity and Stoicism, but it didn't amount to anything.

However, if we skip forward to more modern times, we start to see Stoic ideas gaining traction again and having an influence on a cross-section of different people and fields. Writers, athletes, entrepreneurs, musicians, politicians, psychologists, teachers and countless others are expressing interest in these ideas.

Back in the 1950s, the psychotherapist and psychologist Albert Ellis created a type of therapy called Rational Emotive Behaviour Therapy (REBT). This was heavily influenced by Stoic philosophy. Cognitive Behavioural Therapy (CBT), which was created in the 1960s by the psychiatrist Dr Aaron T. Beck, was also inspired by the Stoics. Yup, both therapies borrow themes and ideas from the Stoics and I'll be referencing these two types of therapy later.

There are many reasons for the resurgence of interest in Stoic philosophy and much comes down to the fact that it's incredibly practical. Life is tough, and Stoicism can help with that.

There is a real online Stoic movement too, as quotes from various Stoic philosophers fill the Internet. Big name and celebrity endorsements also help – when the best-selling author and podcast host Tim Ferriss described Stoicism as his "operating system" for life and talked about how much he loved it, this was wonderful publicity for the philosophy. Tim's passion for Stoicism caused a wave of interest in many of his followers, readers and listeners.

Alongside this are Ryan Holiday's wildly popular Daily Stoic social media accounts. Millions of followers tune in to learn about Stoicism on Instagram, Twitter, Facebook, TikTok, YouTube and via a podcast and newsletter every single day.

There are so many examples of people actually using Stoicism in their lives in the modern era. However, my favourite example comes from a rather unusual place. It's the story of Ross Edgley's groundbreaking swim around Great Britain.

Ross is a British adventure athlete who swam his way into the record books in 2018. Ross spent five months swimming around the entire circumference of Great Britain. That's a whopping 1,791 miles. No one in history has done this before and Ross' account of the swim is phenomenal. He had a support boat where he would sleep each night and he didn't set foot on land for 157 days.

Ross credits Stoic philosophy as being one of the main reasons he was able to complete the swim. Having spent time absorbing the philosophy, he then used the ideas to help him when times got tough. He writes about his experience in his fantastic book *The Art of Resilience*. It's a truly inspirational read with Stoic concepts threaded throughout. He gives wonderful examples of The Stoic Golden Rule in action as he battles tides, encounters wildlife and navigates through blooms of jelly fish.

What I admire most about Ross' Stoic attitude is that he puts his money where his mouth is. Rather than just reading or writing about Stoic philosophy, he's actually putting their ideas into action and using Stoic concepts to help him deal with insanely challenging situations. As Epictetus would say:

"Don't explain your philosophy. Embody it."
Epictetus

This is exactly what Ross has done. What a way to stress-test out a philosophy – swimming around an entire country!

Ross shows us that with the right mindset, we can achieve extraordinary things. Just think about what these Stoic ideas might be able to do for you. Maybe that epic challenge in the back of your mind is achievable after all.

MODERN STOICISM

There might not be a head of the Stoic school or *Stoa Poikile* these days, but there is a growing collective of people interested in these ideas. Writers, athletes, content creators and thinkers are all helping to push the ideas of the Stoics forward. This movement is often referred to as Modern Stoicism. In this movement certain Stoic concepts and ideas have been updated to fit with the modern era – mainly things about Zeus and the gods. As mentioned earlier, it's worth being aware of this as when you read the original Stoics you might become conscious of these tweaks. This will be especially true if you are well versed in the modern Stoic writers and then go back and read the ancient texts.

One of the great things about the modern take on Stoicism is that it continues to grow as the community gets bigger. Stoic ideas will continue to evolve and it's interesting to think about what will come next. With the creation of the Internet, the philosophy now has a global reach. It's wonderful that people from all over the planet are connecting to these ancient concepts. It's an incredibly exciting time for the philosophy.

So, there is my very brief history of Stoicism. We've whizzed through a lot of stuff in a short space of time but hopefully it will have given you a solid grounding and understanding as to where these ideas have come from. And where we are today.

Right, let's crack on with the philosophy and look at some juicy Stoic principles.

PART 2

THE STOIC PRINCIPLES

The following section of the book will look at 10 game-changing ideas from Stoicism. These are the ideas that I've connected with the most from the philosophy and I'm excited to share them with you. All have impacted me in a positive way and on a regular basis. They bring an immense amount of value to my life and have helped me to look at the world in a different way. I'm confident that you will get a lot out of them too.

I would recommend reading them in the order that they appear. Yes, in theory, you could dip in and out of them but as certain ideas build upon each other, it makes sense to read them in sequence.

These principles are all incredibly practical and I encourage you to test them out as you go along. I've created a bunch of exercises for you to try at the end of each principle. Think of these as a call to action – this is where you can put the ideas to the test in the real world. Reading the principles and not using them would be a shame – I believe that these concepts need to be put into practice to be fully understood. It's the pragmatic component of the philosophy that I feel is so important when working with Stoicism.

As a side note – keep your eyes peeled for The Stoic Golden Rule as it threads and weaves its way through these ideas. I'd also encourage you to think about The Cardinal Virtues: Wisdom, Justice, Fortitude, Temperance. Both of these Stoic fundamentals run in the background of Stoic thought. Ask yourself the following questions when working through these principles to help you to relate back to these fundamentals:

1. How does this improve my character? (Cardinal Virtues)
2. What can I *actually* control in this situation? (The Stoic Golden Rule)

Sometimes it will be obvious and you will see how these fundamentals apply to the principles. At other times it might not be so clear. Either way, the goal is to bring a deeper awareness to these principles by having character and control at the forefront of your mind.

It's also worth noting that some of the principles you are about to encounter might seem like common sense. A lot of them have been built on logic and reasoning and are solid ideas. I believe this is why so many people connect with Stoicism. It just makes sense.

So, sit back, relax and get ready for some game-changing philosophy.

3

PRINCIPLE 1:
VOLUNTARY DISCOMFORT

*"We will train both soul and body when
we accustom ourselves to cold, heat, thirst,
hunger, scarcity of food, hardness of bed,
abstaining from pleasures and
enduring pains."*

Musonius Rufus

SUMMARY OF PRINCIPLE

We prepare for adversity by practising adversity.

PRINCIPLE

Voluntary discomfort is one of my favourite Stoic concepts. This was my gateway into the philosophy, so it makes sense to start the principles here. It was the first Stoic idea that I began using in my life – and it really helped my anxiety.

The idea is simple – by deliberately exposing ourselves to hardships, we will be better prepared to face hardships in the future. Essentially, it's training for life. We don't know what's around the corner so preparing ourselves for all sorts of potential adversity is a great insurance policy. By working through deliberate difficulties, we build confidence. We also learn how to cope with challenging situations and develop trust in our ability to get through tough times. It's a powerful concept.

I'm particularly fond of how creative the Stoics were when they applied this idea to their lives. There was a whole cross-section of weird and wonderful things they did to build resilience. Some of these ideas seem bonkers but do make sense when you stop and think about them. For example, the Stoics would sleep on hard surfaces, expose themselves to the cold and the heat, fast from food and water, partake in strenuous exercise, endure pain, skip pleasures, walk barefoot and wear things that would deliberately embarrass them. Essentially, anything that might make them feel uncomfortable would be fully embraced.

This idea was first used by the Cynics (one of the other Ancient Greek Schools of Philosophy) and you can see how it has influenced the Stoics. Diogenes (412–323 BCE), one of the most famous Cynics of all time, used to live in a barrel. Out of choice. He denounced the need for possessions and would regularly defecate in public with no sense of shame. He's quite an extreme example of someone deliberately embracing discomfort. The Cynics would also get naked and hug statues in winter and roll around in hot sand in the summer – something which isn't so popular in modern times. The Stoics borrowed and developed these ideas but never got quite as hardcore as Diogenes. You will find this concept throughout the ancient texts. One of my favourite passages is from Seneca:

"Here's a lesson to test your mind's mettle:
take a part of a week in which you have only
the most meagre and cheap food, dress
scantly in shabby clothes, and ask yourself
if this is really the worst that you feared. It is

> when times are good that you should gird
> yourself for tougher times ahead, for when
> Fortune is kind the soul can build defences
> against her ravages."

Seneca

The whole idea of embracing discomfort was a form of training to the Stoics. It's not supposed to be a masochistic thing (although it might appear to be from the outside). It's there to help us toughen up. It prepares us for the future and to be ready for the challenges that await us.

There are several ways that the Stoics would use this in their lives. I've played around with these ideas and broken them down into themes to give you a general overview of the different types of voluntary discomfort you can try.

DELIBERATE DISCOMFORT

This is pretty straightforward – to expose ourselves to mild discomfort on purpose. The more we do this, the more accustomed to discomfort and/or pain we become. Simple, right?

The most obvious place to seek out mild discomfort is through physical activity. Exercise can certainly be uncomfortable at times, and given the huge variety of physical things we can get our teeth sunk into, we are spoilt for choice. A lot of the Ancient Greeks and Romans were "shredded" – in top physical condition from hard exercise. I mean, just look at the statues! Wrestling was popular among the ancients, and the well-known Latin phrase – "healthy body, healthy mind" (*mens sana in corpore sano*) – shows how important physical exercise was to them. Establishing a long-term relationship with some sort of exercise is great for connecting with this Stoic principle. It's an accessible way to put this theory into practise.

Another popular method of experiencing discomfort is through cold and heat exposure. The Roman Stoic Cato was known for fully embracing the elements. He would stroll around inappropriately dressed for the weather irrespective of the conditions. We can easily apply this in our lives and there are many ways to use temperature and weather exposure to build resilience. In modern Stoic circles the cold shower has become a bit of a cliché and is one of the most common ways to actively practise Stoicism.

Personally, I've had a lot of fun with cold exposure. I've had ice baths, cold baths and done a ton of wild swimming (I live in England so the water is cold all of the time here.) I religiously have a cold shower every day and end up recommending this to everyone I talk to. I've even had a crack at Snowga. What's Snowga, you ask? Simple – snow + yoga. Lots of Stoic boxes got ticked when I tried this out in my garden. My neighbours also got to witness me rolling around half-naked in the snow on the coldest day of the year ... That must have been a strange sight for them!

When it comes to heat exposure, the sauna is a popular option. Lots of cultures use a combination of cold water followed by the hot sauna as a way to invigorate the body. (I think this goes without saying, but be careful in the sauna – pushing yourself can be extremely dangerous.)

Embracing the elements is another way to explore all of this. If it starts raining, why not go for a walk? I absolutely love rainy runs. If the conditions are rough, I know it's going to be a character-building experience. However, this backfired on me when I went for a run during the "storm of the century". Storm Ciara hit the UK with 90mph winds and I thought it would be a great training opportunity. It was a terrible idea ... The wind was so strong that I could barely breathe and ended up almost stuck on top of an exposed hill. Then, a flying branch nearly fell on my head. I guess the moral of the story is to find the balance with your resilience training and not get yourself killed.

The other classic Stoic deliberate discomfort exercise is to sleep on the floor without a pillow, duvet or mattress. This is hardcore. After spending a night sleeping on the ground, a bed has a new level of comfort. I can attest to this. If I spend the night sleeping on the floor next to my bed, I am *incredibly* grateful for my mattress.

There are many other ways to seek out physical discomfort – why not try avoiding painkillers when facing mild pain, ordering an acupressure bed of nails mat and spending time on it, holding different stress positions, or throwing a load of Lego on the floor and walking over it. There are so many things you can do. The main goal, though, should be to get stuck in and actually test this idea out in the real world.

"SHAME-ATTACKING"

Embarrassment is another way to experience mental discomfort. Cato (him again) was known for wearing clothes that would make his peers laugh at him. He would deliberately do this to practise feeling shame and to then overcome it.

I love this idea. I'm an introvert so the thought of deliberately wearing something ridiculous makes me feel extremely uncomfortable. This is hard for me to do. Therefore, it's a *great* thing for me to do.

To explore this idea, I bought a series of weird hats from Japan … By wearing these hats in public, it's easy to feel like an idiot. I've demonstrated these hats in my workshops on Stoicism and, without a shadow of a doubt, everyone's favourite is the crab hat. Yes, it's a hat that looks like a crab. Yes, it's utterly preposterous. But that's the point. By embracing the things that make us feel embarrassed, we become better at feeling comfortable in our own skin. Don't just take mine or Cato's word for it though ...

This technique is known as "shame-attacking" and is used in REBT therapy to help patients deal with social anxiety. Shame-attacking exposes patients to situations where they will feel uncomfortable in order for them to learn to relax in those situations. This process is called desensitization.

Albert Ellis, the creator of REBT therapy, was known for his sense of humour and had fun with this concept. A famous exercise he would get his patients to do was to take a pet banana for a walk through a busy public space. By the way, a "pet banana" is literally just a banana tied to a piece of string. The internal fear of being judged by others is challenged by this whole process. Without an explanation, this act can look rather unusual and can make you feel extremely self-conscious ... It's a successful way to build confidence and you can see how this was inspired by the Stoics.

The other thing Ellis would encourage his patients to do was to behave in an embarrassing way in public. For example – singing out loud while walking down the street, yawning obnoxiously when someone is telling a story or asking really stupid questions. Personally, I like the idea of going into a bookstore and asking if they sell air-conditioning units. I definitely think there's room to be creative with this idea.

The list of ways to embarrass ourselves and test out shame-attacking is endless, but it's important to note that all of these exercises should focus on us being uncomfortable and are not supposed to be cruel to other people. So, if you decide to come up with some of your own socially awkward experiments, don't forget to make yourself the butt of the joke.

Why not test out this idea by going for a barefoot stroll while singing to yourself in a busy place? You could always take along a pet banana if you don't fancy doing it alone. I'm sure the Stoics would approve.

DELIBERATE DEPRIVATION

Another popular way the Stoics would engage in voluntary discomfort would be through deliberate deprivation. This is pretty much what it says on the tin: to deliberately avoid something that you want or like. Not as a punishment but as a test of self-control and mental strength.

The classic example is fasting from food or water (get advice from a medical professional if you decide to emulate the Stoics with this one). By depriving themselves of food and water, the Stoics could practise managing the discomfort of cravings within their bodies. A lot of modern Stoics employ intermittent fasting as part of their practice.

But it doesn't have to be as extreme as fasting, and the simple act of skipping treats like desserts and sauces can tick the box. The Stoic Musonius Rufus was a big fan of simplistic eating and living. He emphasized the importance of being able to have self-discipline when it comes to food. Rufus saw food as the perfect opportunity to exercise self-control. Not overeating, along with a simple and clean diet, was his recommendation for living a good life. I'm confident he would go into a state of shock if he saw how much tomato ketchup I use on stuff. Something for me to work on …

Turning down that glass of wine, pint of beer or half gallon of ketchup can be a way to put this whole concept into practise. Again, don't see this as negative, it is an exercise in cultivating resilience. By refraining from excess, we can appreciate what we do have. Developing an appreciation for the simpler things in life has many benefits.

Deliberate deprivation also works well in the tech world. Ideas like digital fasting (where you spend time away from technology) and social media fasting (where you keep off social media) is a brilliant way to apply this concept to modern life. So many people are addicted to their phones and find spending time away from the screen mentally uncomfortable. I know how tough this can be and have personally struggled with this at times – the screen time feature on my phone is both shocking and helpful. The amount of time I spend on certain apps is highlighted by this feature and it's alarming how quickly those minutes stack up. By deliberately setting restrictions on our tech use, we can put this ancient Stoic practice to the test.

There are so many ways to deprive ourselves of pleasure. But always remember, this is in the name of mental training and is not a punishment.

FAILURE AND REJECTION INOCULATION

Strictly speaking, this isn't something the Stoics would do, but it's an excellent practice to develop the idea of voluntary discomfort in the modern world. It works the same way as being inoculated against disease – by exposing your body to a small amount of the virus, you learn how to deal with it. Just replace "virus" with "failure and rejection". In deliberately seeking out situations where we are likely to fail or be rejected, we get better at dealing with those experiences. We learn how to handle rejection and failure by facing them head-on. There's nothing like direct experience for teaching us a valuable lesson.

For some people, a fear of failure or a negative response can be an incredibly paralysing force, preventing them from trying new things, meeting new people or doing anything to stand out from the crowd. Similar to the REBT shame-attacking exercise, failure and rejection inoculation can help to manage that force.

For example, try asking for ridiculous requests when ordering a pizza. Call up and ask for a square pizza. You might feel a bit silly, but that's the point! You could even spice things up further by asking for a special message or drawing in the top of the pizza box. Remember that the purpose of this exercise is to fail and get rejected. Ultimately, it's about paying attention to how you feel while requesting the square pizza and to get comfortable asking for things with an uncertain outcome.

It's a harmless exercise but builds confidence if you do it enough. And why not ask for a discount while you're at it? There's absolutely nothing wrong with asking for a discount but it can make us feel socially awkward – a great thing!

To play with this idea more, try to get a selfie with a complete stranger. It's a pretty weird thing to ask someone that you don't know, and the chance of getting rejected is high. The less explaining you do up front, the harder it becomes!

Please note that all of this does come with a warning – some of these exercises will work and you won't fail or get rejected. This can actually be very funny. You might end up with a square pizza or a little discount. These are a nice bonus, but technically you will have failed as the point of the exercise is to fail in your request. You can get some great stories trying out these exercises though. For a little inspiration, take a peek at the American series *Impractical Jokers*. Some of the challenges they complete are uncomfortable to watch.

A NAVY SEAL'S GUIDE TO VOLUNTARY DISCOMFORT

One of my favourite examples of voluntary discomfort in the modern world is documented in the fantastic book *Living with a SEAL: 31 Days Training with the Toughest Man on the Planet* by Jesse Itzler. Jesse decided that it would be an interesting experiment to invite the former Navy SEAL David Goggins to come and live with him for a month. The reason – to help Jesse build resilience. If you know anything about Goggins, you know that Jesse was bold to do this. Goggins has gained worldwide recognition as one of the toughest people on the planet. He's known for ultra-endurance racing, motivational speeches, has a pull-up world record (4,030 pull-ups in 24 hours) and a best-selling book. He was also part of the elite Navy SEALs and exemplifies discipline and resilience. His list of achievements is impressive.

Goggins spent a month living with Jesse and gave him a crash course in voluntary discomfort. He got Jesse doing things that he didn't think he was capable of, from smashing out hundreds of pull-ups to icy lake dips to sleeping on a wooden chair. Goggins was there pushing Jesse to do crazy things all day every day. At first, Jesse found himself way out of his depth, but over time his confidence and resilience increased. He has fantastic anecdotes from the whole experience and as Jesse has a family with small children, having a SEAL live with all of them led to some funny situations. The results after a month of living with a SEAL were significant with regards to Jesse's mindset, and he speaks highly of the experiment.

We don't have to invite an ex-Navy SEAL to come and live with us to use this Stoic principle in our lives (although that would be quite an experience). In reality, there are lots of ways to explore the idea of voluntary discomfort. Any time we step outside of our comfort zones, we are putting this principle into action.

The anti-bucket list fits perfectly here. By exposing ourselves to our fears, we can learn to manage/overcome them. Fear exposure is an incredible way to build resilience and a great addition to your Stoic training.

FINAL THOUGHTS

Modern life is often geared toward making us as comfortable as possible. We have air-conditioning in case we get too hot. We have heating in case we get too cold. We have takeaways, fast food, Internet shopping and same-day-delivery. We have soft mattresses with quilts and fabric softener that makes our clothes smell crisp and fresh. There is a whole host of things that have been designed to make our lives more convenient and more comfortable. It has become easier and easier for us to avoid discomfort – but is this really helping us? If we aren't accustomed to any discomfort at all, we can end up complaining too quickly when things get tough. Even the slightest setback or mildest discomfort can cause us to throw our figurative toys out of the pram. This is exactly what this Stoic principle is training us to avoid.

I have some specific exercises coming up that you can use to begin your journey with voluntary discomfort. So, when you find yourself in an intense situation that was totally self-inflicted, remember Seneca's wise words:

"So it is that soldiers practice manoeuvres in peacetime, erecting bunkers with no enemies in sight and exhausting themselves under no attack so that when it comes they won't grow tired."
Seneca

PRACTICAL EXERCISES

The purpose of the following exercises is to build resilience and create a mindset that can handle adversity.

ANTI-BUCKET LIST
Create your own anti-bucket list and write down the things that you fear. Now think about how you can turn these fears into challenges. If you're afraid of heights, go and book a

climbing session. Terrified of needles, then sign up to give blood. For more details, revisit my introduction to this idea on page xvii.

DELIBERATE DISCOMFORT

1. Start an exercise routine. This can be anything you want but remember that physical exercise is a great way to train resilience. If you already have a regular routine, explore new types of exercise and play around with the length and intensity of your workouts.
2. Embrace cold water. Take a cold shower or cold bath, go wild swimming or treat yourself to an ice bath.
3. Get creative and come up with interesting ways to make yourself uncomfortable. Bonus points awarded for bizarre ideas! Remember the Lego-walk?

SHAME-ATTACKING

1. Take your pet banana or pet vegetable for a walk in a busy place. My preference would be a vegetable. Why? Well, I guess it's a bit more durable than a banana ... either way you're probably going to feel like an idiot (just what we want).
2. Go for a barefoot walk in a public place.
3. Sing to yourself while walking down a busy street.

DELIBERATE DEPRIVATION

1. Drink only water for one week – no tea/coffee/ juice/alcohol, etc.
2. Deprive yourself of social media and TV for 48 hours.
3. Ban sweet treats for one week (basically, avoid anything sugary).

Please note: All of these can be made harder by extending the length of time to a month or a year.

FAILURE AND REJECTION INOCULATION

1. Order a square pizza.
2. Ask for a discount on the next item you buy (irrespective of what it is and where you happen to be).
3. Try and get a selfie of you and a stranger.

JOURNALING PROMPTS

Your journaling exercise for this principle is a combination of list making and reviewing around the practical exercises. Start by creating your anti-bucket list, which can be an ongoing exercise that you add to over time. This warrants a lot of thought, so don't rush it.

Next, write reflectively on each exercise. How did the cold shower go? What about the pet vegetable walk? Did you actually do it? How did you feel? Which vegetable did you choose? Or did you stick with the banana? You could even share your experiences online as a way to engage with the Stoic community. I'm confident that others would be interested to hear about your adventures with voluntary discomfort. I know I would love to hear how you got on with it. In fact, come and say hi on Instagram and tell me all about it! My handle is @dothingsthatchallengeyou.

Think about the types of voluntary discomfort you can bring into your life on a regular basis. Creating a list of potential ideas for this is a good way to come up with an interesting to-do list. The bolder, the better, I say!

4

PRINCIPLE 2: PERCEPTION

*"It isn't the things themselves that
disturb people, but the judgements that
they form about them."*

Epictetus

SUMMARY OF PRINCIPLE

We have to pay careful attention to our minds and their ability to
turn mountains into molehills and molehills into mountains. We
live our lives according to our judgements of the external world.

PRINCIPLE

The Stoics had a lot to say about our perceptions and I've
personally found their ideas to be very helpful in my life. Having
first-hand experience of how powerful the mind can be, I am
acutely aware of how my thinking affects my reality.

When I was experiencing severe anxiety and panic attacks
I had problems with viewing the world objectively. Everything
felt like it was about to go wrong. I would worry that the worst-
case scenario was always around the corner and I had a

tendency to label a lot of stuff as "terrible" or "disastrous" when it really wasn't. This extreme judgement of everything caused serious problems for me.

For example, I remember taking a wrong turn in the car during the peak of my anxiety and practically melting down over the situation. I got into a real flap and started to panic about having made a mistake. I wasn't being clear with my thinking. All I needed to do was find somewhere to turn the car around. It really wasn't a problem but my mind was judging it differently and labelling it as catastrophic.

The Stoic answer to all of this is to seek objectivity in the way we think – to view things as they are, rather than adding a biased running commentary to the situation. It's all too easy to make things worse by overthinking or catastrophizing. I'm sure you can spot everyday examples in your life where something small is blown out of proportion. It's easy for us to do this, especially when we're in an anxious mental space.

Any one of us can freak out over an incorrectly made coffee or a queue, and the smallest problems can easily be seen as disasters. It's when we encounter this negative thinking that we really need to lean into objectivity. Unfortunately, it isn't always easy.

Human beings are great at judging things in a negative way; it's in our genetic make-up. Evolutionary science suggests that the human brain tends to have a negative disposition as this is a very effective survival mechanism. Back in the day (when we used to live in caves), we were always on the lookout for what might potentially kill us. Is that Steve in the bushes or is it some giant hungry cat? The more paranoid the mind, the less likely we were to find ourselves caught off guard. That brain is still with us, along with its judgy mindset, and this can be problematic in modern life. So, if you are naturally pessimistic at times, don't beat yourself up – this is a survival skill that has kept the human race alive for a long time.

Having said all of this, the Stoics strived to face everything in an objective, not a negative, manner. They paid careful attention to impressions and judgements to not let negative emotions rule their thinking.

For example, when it pours with rain, as it often does in England, saying that the weather is *terrible* or *rubbish* is a judgement. It's not an objective statement. When it rains, it's just rain. The fact that we think it sucks is our problem. The rain is outside of our control and a natural part of life. If it never rained, we would have other issues to deal with (and we could easily complain about these too).

The Stoic Golden Rule – we can't control what happens to us, but we can control our response – and perception go hand in hand. If we fully understand this rule, it can have a profound effect on how we view reality. There are so many things that we can't influence, so judging them harshly can make our lives unpleasant and lead to all sorts of problems.

Working with The Stoic Golden Rule has massively helped me to work on my perceptions. When I encounter a situation that my mind perceives to be negative, I focus on this rule. Reminding myself that I can't control the traffic, the weather or the speed at which other people walk helps me to avoid getting worked up about those things. Granted, I'm not always perfect at doing this (just ask my wife) but having a strategy makes me a lot better.

The Stoics suggest that we play it cool and remain as objective as possible to everything that happens to us. It's the labels that we add to everything that can cause us problems. Aurelius puts it like this:

"If you are pained by any external thing, it is not this thing that disturbs you, but your own judgement about it. And it is in your power to wipe out this judgement now."

Marcus Aurelius

By becoming conscious of how much we judge everything, we can start to challenge this thinking. Modern psychology has a lot to say on all of this ...

JUDGEMENTS AND PERCEPTION IN MODERN PSYCHOLOGY

There are two types of therapy in the modern world that I think are great for helping us to work on our judgements and perceptions. These are Cognitive Behavioural Therapy (CBT) and Neuro Linguistic Programming (NLP). The first focuses on questioning our thoughts and perceptions and the second more on the words we use.

In CBT, we are encouraged to investigate our thoughts about things. When we have a negative thought about something, we are urged to whip out the logic-hose and spray the thought with logic and reasoning. OK, I made up the term logic-hose but I think it fits well. Imagine you're trying to put out a fire (negative thinking) with a hose (that sprays logic). The more you question your negative or troublesome thoughts, the better you get at weighting them in reality and not automatically believing every thought that comes into your head.

For example, if you're strolling along and suddenly trip up a curb, your brain might say to you – "You're an idiot! Why did you fall over?" This isn't helpful, but by using logic, you can fight back against the thought. You might respond to the negativity by questioning yourself – "Am I really an idiot for tripping up a curb? No. I just need to pay more attention to what I'm doing. Everyone makes mistakes."

If you push back on negative thinking or unhelpful assumptions frequently enough, it can make a huge difference to how you handle that internal dialogue. As I mentioned earlier, CBT was influenced by Stoicism and you can see how questioning our judgements about things is such an important factor here. The Stoics loved reason so would value this type of internal inquiry. The Socratic dialogue of questioning everything can work wonders in our minds.

NLP is slightly different and gets us to pay attention to the actual words we use (both internally and externally). A classic example might be replacing the word *have* with *get* in the following sentence: "I have to go to the gym." This then becomes: "I get to go to the gym."

Have sounds like we are being forced to do something whereas *get* feels like a choice. It's a subtle difference but helps to frame the situation constructively.

By changing various words, especially internally, we begin to alter the way we interact with and view the world. It takes time and practise but by changing the architecture of our internal dialogue, we can empower ourselves to think differently.

Words can be extremely powerful so we need to pay close attention to those we use. There's a wonderful TED talk by Lera Boroditsky called "How Language Shapes the Way We Think", about how different languages make us perceive the world in different ways. She talks about how our language can influence how we interact with the world, and gives a fascinating example of an Aboriginal community in Australia that don't use left or right in their language. For them, everything is based on cardinal directions – north, east, south and west. So, this tribe would say things like, "There's an ant on your south-east leg." They also greet each other by asking which direction they are going. Instead of, "Hi Margaret, how are you today?" they would say, "Margaret, which way are you going? North-east, again?" OK, maybe that's not the exact wording they would use, but hopefully you get what I mean. Can you imagine how that would work in the West ... "Er, hold on while I check my phone!"

The fact that this tribe constantly use direction in their language means that they know what direction they are facing at all times. If the language you use has the power to keep you orientated, what do you think will happen if you keep using negative words to yourself? It can completely change your perception on reality. Your mindset will start to reflect the words you choose.

EXILE

Let's look at a practical example of the Stoics dealing with something that most people would perceive as a "bad" situation: exile.

The Stoics seemed to get themselves exiled left, right and centre. By living lives of strict moral integrity, they would end up with enemies. They were known for seeking social justice and speaking out against authority if they felt something wasn't right. (Justice was one of their cardinal virtues, after all). As you can imagine, this didn't always end well. If you were doing something that the powers that be were annoyed with, it was easy to receive a death sentence or banishment to somewhere well out of the way.

Seneca, Epictetus, Rufus and a handful of other Stoic philosophers were all exiled at some point in their lives, but the Stoics had an interesting perception of the situation ... Their belief was that the environment wasn't the problem. You could still live a virtuous life and be a decent person even when forced into an inhospitable or undesirable environment. In fact, Rufus pointed out that exile can be good for people. Living a simple life, especially if exiled somewhere lacking luxury and resources, can help people to overcome "soft living". As long as we have the essentials to survive, we can thrive by working on our virtues and character. Given that Rufus was exiled to a tiny, arid and desolate island called Gyaros (the choice of exile for the most vile criminals in the times of the Roman Empire), he was pretty qualified to comment on all of this. No back-seat philosophizing there!

We have a choice about how we view any situation. If we can't control it, we have to change the way we think about it. The Stoics viewed exile as an "indifferent" – something that they would probably prefer not to happen but they could handle it if it did. And if they had to handle it, they would choose their response to the situation:

> "I must go into exile. Does any man then hinder me from going with smiles and cheerfulness and contentment?"
>
> Epictetus

LOCKDOWN

Exile is something that doesn't really exist in modern life. Being a refugee might be the closest thing we have. The Stoics wrote a lot about exile but this was never something that I thought would be that relevant to me. However, it took on a different colour during the COVID-19 global pandemic. Suddenly these words had a new depth to them. The way the Stoics handled exile was something that certainly helped me during lockdown.

As the virus ripped through the population and caused death and economic destruction, a large percentage of the world were forced into various types of lockdown, ranging from very strict to more lenient. Obviously, this isn't the same as being thrown out of your home and banished to some far away destination, but there are similarities. Firstly, this was completely outside of our control. When the Stoics were sent into exile, it wasn't what they had chosen to do either. Secondly, we were stuck in one place and our movements were restricted. Our geographic limitations meant that our worlds had become small, just as when some of the Stoics were sent to remote islands.

My journey with lockdown was interesting. I certainly felt cooped up and frustrated by everything. However, I was incredibly grateful to still be working (Zoom became the new normal) and my friends and family were all healthy, so I was very lucky.

I wanted to make the best out of the situation and was inspired by how the Stoics handled exile. Their perceptions of something that a lot of people considered terrible made me reconsider what I was dealing with. Working with this philosophy helped me to handle a very tough situation. In fact, it helped me to remain objective when it felt like the world was ending.

CHALLENGING OUR PERCEPTIONS

Doing things that we think are going to be boring, difficult or frustrating is a great way to get an insight into our perceptions and automatic judgements. If we pay close attention to our minds while doing them, we learn a lot from these experiences. Seeking out things that are likely to trigger these automatic judgements within us is perfect for training our minds. I have a few things you can try to test out your perceptions.

The first is a quick and easy food-based way to challenge your thinking and perceptions: pick something that you used to hate eating as a child and try it. For me, I used to have a massive problem with leek and potato soup – the fibres from the leek always made me think there was hair in my soup. I'm sure you have many examples of gross food from your childhood. When you've conjured up those memories, seek out that food ... Is it as bad as you remember? Could you eat it for several days in a row? If not, why not? To take it further, why not seek out something that you know is going to taste disgusting and eat it?

I do this exercise a lot and enjoy pushing myself to try different foods. I wrote about my experience of eating durian fruit in my first book (it didn't go well) but have continued to use this exercise in my life. It's a great way to challenge my perceptions. Right now, I'm eating a lot of celery. I try to be objective while I eat it because I really dislike the taste. I treat it as a mindful exercise and explore the flavour – I still think it's gross. Another example is Marmite. My wife, Helen, loves Marmite but I hate it. This is something that I also keep coming back to as I know I dislike it. I often find that my perceived dislike for a flavour is worse than the actual reality.

A second way to challenge your perceptions is music-based. By actively listening to a genre of music that you dislike or think you will dislike, you have the perfect opportunity to try objective listening. What is objective listening? It's simply sitting and listening to something without running a commentary on the music. You simply listen. It's actually harder than it sounds.

The specific album that I recommend you listen to is *The Olatunji Concert: The Last Live Recording* by John Coltrane. It's pure chaotic noise and, if you haven't ever heard Free Jazz before, you'll be in for a surprise. Most people struggle to listen to this album and remain objective about it. Typically, people can't relate to it as music because it's so abstract and think that it sounds "bad". Someone once told me that the album "sounded like an elephant dying". Give it a try and pay attention to your thoughts throughout the experience.

It's worth noting that I chose this album because I know it's considered hard to listen to. John Coltrane is my favourite Jazz musician and his album *Blue Train* is a go-to for me while writing. I love his music and although I've recommended *The Olatunji Concert* as a challenge, it comes from a place of love and deep respect for his work.

There are tons of other things you can do to invoke potential negative judgements. Just think of something rubbish and go

HOW TO CONTROL THE UNCONTROLLABLE

and do it. For example – watching TV shows or movies that you know you will dislike, going to places that you think look boring and trying activities in which you have no interest. While you're doing this, pay close attention to your mind. See if you find yourself complaining or being negative in your judgements about everything ...

COMPLAINING

How often do you complain about things? Do you regularly unload your complaints onto others? It's interesting to think about this.

Complaining is essentially us negatively judging a situation and then sharing our thoughts with anyone who will listen. And if no one is around, we end up complaining to ourselves. Tutting and sighing audibly is the perfect example of someone complaining to themselves in their head. Rather than say anything, they release a noise, but we all know what this noise means.

The truth is, it's easy for us to moan about things, especially when they don't go our way. There will always be things to complain about so a healthy response to the urge to complain is to focus our energy on what we can do about the situation rather than sit there in a stink. The Stoics advised against complaining:

"Don't be overheard complaining ... Not even to yourself."
Marcus Aurelius

FINAL THOUGHTS

Our minds determine the kind of experience we have on this planet so it makes sense to become conscious of our thoughts about things. According to the Stoics, we should strive to pay attention to our judgements and fight to remain objective in our behaviour.

A lot of modern therapies encourage us to cultivate this type of thinking. The mind is incredibly powerful so we must use it in a way that helps us to thrive. If we apply logic and reasoning, we have a solid foundation for everything we do. How we choose to see the world has a humungous impact on our lives. Our thinking creates our reality.

So ... Pay attention to your mind and remember Aurelius' important advice:

> "The soul becomes dyed with the colour of its thoughts."
>
> Marcus Aurelius

PRACTICAL EXERCISES

The purpose of these exercises is to help you view the world objectively.

BECOME OBJECTIVE

The next time you find yourself stuck in traffic, on a delayed train or queuing, focus on being objective. Remember the logic-hose?! Well, start spraying! Alternatively, pretend that you're a robot and are completely objective to everything that you are experiencing. Let the situation unfold without judging it. Say to yourself, "I am now stuck in traffic." Do not add a "and it's terrible/I'm going to be late" bit – fight to view everything purely objectively. Stick to the facts and don't add labels or predict future doom. You can expand this exercise by applying it to every situation you face, or every difficult person you encounter or anything that doesn't go "your way". Try to remain objective when things don't go to plan or you encounter negativity.

CHALLENGE YOUR PERCEPTIONS
1. Eat something that you don't like.
2. Listen to *The Olatunji Concert: The Last Live Recording* by John Coltrane.
3. Create a list of things that you think will be boring – now go and do them.

SELF-IMPOSED MINI-EXILE
Set a timer for an hour and lock yourself in a room without any entertainment. No phone. No computer. No book, etc. Literally sit there and do nothing. The goal with this exercise is to observe your thinking while completing your mini-exile. Pay particular attention to your internal dialogue and look for negative impressions and judgements. When the timer rings, make notes.

   *This exercise can be made harder by doing it somewhere ridiculous. A cupboard? The garden shed? Under your bed? You have options.

NLP AND CBT
Investigate these two types of modern psychology – maybe watch a couple of YouTube videos or put a book or two on your TBR (to be read) list. Unpackage the concepts a little more and make notes on the ideas you like the most.

THE COMPLAINT JAR
I've created a little exercise to help with complaining. This is also a great way to become aware of your perceptions. It's called the "Complaint Jar" and it's easy to use. Each time you catch yourself complaining about something, you have to add

a token to a jar. You can simply put small pieces of paper into a glass for this and it doesn't have to be anything fancy.

At the end of the week, count up how many pieces of paper you have in your glass. This number represents an amount of money that you will lose. I recommend deciding how much each complaint is worth before you start this exercise; for example, one piece of paper equals a penny, a pound or a dollar, etc. You decide.

You must then donate this money to a charity of your choice. Or, if you really want an incentive to not lose the money (because let's face it, donating money to a charity is a positive thing), you can select a cause that you disagree with and donate the money there. A political party that you despise is a good incentive. If you know that every complaint you make will essentially donate money to a cause you hate, it'll make you VERY conscious about complaining.

You might decide for the Complaint Jar to only be for verbal complaints at first. But as you get better, you can add to it each time you complain to yourself in your head.

JOURNALING PROMPTS

Your main journaling exercise for this principle is to build awareness of your perceptions. Each time you pre-emptively judge a situation, make a mental note. Record this in your journal and compare your initial impression of the situation with the reality. How did things actually play out in the end? Was it as bad as you thought it would be? Or was it worse? Start collecting these moments. Remember, awareness of first impressions allows you to challenge unhelpful ones.

You can also reflectively write on the exercises in this principle. How did you find *The Olatunji Concert* by John Coltrane? Maybe list some genres of music that you dislike and listen to them objectively. Write down what you thought of each song. Pay attention to the mind throughout.

What about the food exercise? How did that go? List foods that you dislike and write about your experience eating them.

Did you have a go at being a robot? Did you manage to remain objective in traffic? What about your mini-exile? How did that go?

5

PRINCIPLE 3: SETBACKS

"Just as nature takes every obstacle, every impediment, and works around it – turns it to its purposes, incorporates it into itself – so, too, a rational being can turn each setback into raw material and use it to achieve its goal."

Marcus Aurelius

SUMMARY OF PRINCIPLE

Things will go wrong and we will face setbacks. Learning to embrace these difficulties can change our lives in an empowering way.

PRINCIPLE

Stuff goes wrong all the time and setbacks are an inevitable part of being human. Just spend a moment thinking about the last time something went wrong in your life – you likely won't have to think for long.

One minute you're working out in your front room, the next minute your radiator blows a cap and starts spraying boiling hot water all over your house ... One minute you're sightseeing in Taiwan and slip down a two-inch step, the next minute you have a back injury that takes six months to heal ... One minute you're queuing calmly in traffic, the next minute a drunk driver crashes their car into the back of yours ...

All of these things happened to me. Yes, they are bizarre examples of things going wrong but I can assure you this is barely scratching the surface. I could fill multiple books with setbacks. We all could!

Every single one of us has faced countless setbacks in our lives. From minor inconveniences to epic disasters, volumes of prose could be written about the challenges humanity has had to collectively face. This is the way the world works.

We all have to face difficult circumstances in life and there's no escaping this fact. Some people will have to deal with absolutely brutal setbacks whereas others will have it a bit easier. Life can be unpredictable.

So, what can we do? Well, the Stoics have an answer that we've already looked at – The Dichotomy of Control. Yes, The Stoic Golden Rule again. By focusing on how we respond to external situations (setbacks in this case), we put the power back in our hands. By taking charge of the situation, we can proactively deal with the cards we have been dealt. We might not have willingly wanted things to turn out this way, but we can respond philosophically, and thrive despite the circumstances.

One of my favourite sayings on all of this is by Jon Kabat-Zinn, the internationally-renowned mindfulness teacher and scientist:

"You can't stop the waves, but you can learn to surf."

Jon Kabat-Zinn

Although Jon is not a Stoic (as far as I'm aware), he sums up how, even though life keeps hitting us with challenges, we can do something about it. We can learn to face these difficulties and obstacles and actually thrive as we gracefully handle the difficult times in life.

The Stoics were also firm believers that we can handle setbacks with finesse and even grow to love them ... Yup, we can learn to enjoy it when things don't go to plan.

AMOR FATI

The Stoic concept of *amor fati* is particularly relevant when dealing with setbacks. The expression means "a love of fate". The term is relatively new and you won't find it in the ancient texts. In Modern Stoicism it's used to express the Stoic attitude of embracing what happens to us. Epictetus puts it beautifully:

"Don't seek for everything to happen as you wish it would, but rather wish that everything happens as it actually will – then your life will flow well."

Epictetus

The goal is to actually love what happens to us, irrespective of what that is. Obviously, it's a lot easier to say this than to put it into practice. I mean, it's hard to rejoice when things go wrong – "Yippee, I just pulled off the door handle," or, "Hurray, I've just broken my leg." Thinking like this is a big ask, but being able to embrace whatever happens to us can change our relationship with these events. When we accept that we have little control over what happens to us, we accept things more openly. And really, acceptance is the first step in being able to work with what's in front of us.

Amor fati is all about thriving when facing setbacks. A love of fate and what happens to us is a very Stoic attitude to adopt indeed. It might feel counter-intuitive to lean into things when they go wrong, but embracing the challenges with the right mindset can make a world of difference.

DEALING WITH SETBACKS

When dealing with setbacks, it's extremely important to have the right attitude toward the situation. Our attitudes determine the type of outcome we get so we need to be careful with our thinking – remember the Perception principle! If we start sulking and thinking catastrophically, it's hard to handle the situation effectively. More stuff can go wrong and we can end up in a right mess.

There are two effective ways to handle setbacks that I love using in my life. They are excellent at helping me to work with a challenging situation and I highly recommend that you test them out in the real world. The first is based on The Stoic Golden Rule, and the second is about how we frame the situation we find ourselves in.

WHAT CAN I CONTROL?

When something goes wrong, the first thing I try to do is think about what I can actually control in the situation. This thinking may take a minute or two, but it's totally worth it. I run through all of the things outside of my control and all of the things within my control. I then come up with a plan of action. The more often I do this, the better I get at it. Sometimes this technique is quick to use and it just comes naturally. At other times I have to work hard to list everything and trudge through all of my options. If I'm facing a particularly big problem and I have time, I will actually write a "control list" and use this as a springboard for a plan of action. This makes a BIG difference to how I view the situation.

For example, I once found myself stuck on a train coming into London. The weather had been horrific and there were severe problems because of this (good old England!). My train was half underground and half above ground and it didn't move for two hours. We all ended up being evacuated along the tracks. This made me incredibly late for an important event. This is something that had the potential to really stress me out … I'm one of those people who thinks that if I'm on time, I'm actually late. I always like to arrive early. Yes, it drives my wife Helen mad. Anyway, focusing on what I could actually control in this situation really helped me to have command over my mind and not fixate on the fact that I was going to be late. I couldn't control the situation – but I could control my response.

Getting stuck on a train is certainly the kind of thing that would have made me incredibly panicky in the past. Focusing on The Stoic Golden Rule was helpful and allowed me to feel somewhat proactive about the situation, even though I wasn't going anywhere fast. I sent some emails, made a few calls and tried to treat the situation as a Stoic test. This worked wonders.

Knowing what I can and can't control allows me to put my energy in the right place. This, in turn, helps me to create a specific plan based on the situation at hand. Having a plan is powerful and enables me to know where my attention and focus should be. This feels both proactive and effective. I find that the act of doing something can really help me to feel like I'm addressing the problem. Procrastination can make things worse when dealing with a setback.

OK, granted – sometimes the best option when dealing with a setback is to wait things out and be patient. However, knowing that this is the best plan (after having run through all of my options) makes it easier to be passive and wait out the storm. Realizing that it's outside of my control means I can accept the situation for what it is.

REFRAMING

Reframing a situation is all about altering the way we view the world. There are some real parallels with the Perception principle here – how what we think determines our reality. So, by changing the way we think, we change how we experience a setback. We just need to think about the setback in a different light. Simple.

There are many ways we can view problems/obstacles and I'll give you a few options to play around with here. The following examples encourage you to view what you are experiencing with different mindsets. Test them out in difficult situations and see which are helpful.

THE COMEDY MINDSET

Look for the humour in a situation and think about how this setback would be used in a stand-up comedy set. See if you can build jokes off the back of what you are experiencing. Humour can be powerful and help take the sting out of an unpleasant situation.

THE HERO MINDSET

Imagine that you are the protagonist in a novel or movie and this is an obstacle that you have to heroically overcome. What actions would you heroically take to deal with the situation?

THE WRITER MINDSET

Look for how this could be great material for your blog or article. Imagine that you've been commissioned by a newspaper to describe your setback. How would you view it then? This is something that I use a lot. I find that when something doesn't go to plan, I can often use the material to illustrate a point in my writing or on social media.

THE STOIC MINDSET

Imagine that you are going to handle the setback like a true Stoic legend. How would you do that? The exercise in the Role Models principle – *What Would the Stoics Do?* – might be handy here (Principle 5).

THE CREATIVE MINDSET

When dealing with a difficult setback, try to come up with the most innovative and creative solution possible. The crazier, the better! They say that necessity is the mother of invention. Well, get creating and see if you can come up with a solution to what you are facing.

I try to use all of the above mindsets as much as possible when managing a setback. They all work differently so sometimes I'll have to cycle through a few to find the one that works best for the situation I'm facing.

One of my favourite examples of using a creative mindset to handle a problem was when I was off-roading in the Colorado Rocky Mountains with my friend Matt. Determined to test out his new beast of a truck, Matt had chosen a remote off-road route that would take us to a beautiful lake high in the mountains. The only issue was that Matt's truck was big and the track we were driving along was pretty narrow. When I say "pretty narrow", I'm talking a few inches either side of each wing mirror. All was well and good until several miles along this track we encountered an obstacle – two giant boulders blocking the way. If you had a normal-sized vehicle, you would be able to drive between the boulders. But the truck was far too big to get through. It seemed like the only option was to turn around. But there was nowhere to turn around. Reversing miles down the narrow lane wouldn't work either. The turning circle of the truck meant that it was extremely difficult to do this. So, we were stuck. And I instantly became worried about bears!

I'm not going to lie, it was insanely stressful and we weren't feeling great about the situation. It was scary. But, we had to get on with things and getting caught up in worry wasn't helping.

We eventually came up with an over-the-top and ambitious plan – building a ramp with all of the loose rocks lying around. The ramp would mean that the truck's right wheels would go over the boulder on the right-hand side of the track. After an intense hour or so of building the ramp we tested it out and it worked. Creativity saved us! The Creative Mindset allowed us to handle the situation effectively.

EVERYTHING'S A CHALLENGE

Another great way to view setbacks is by seeing them as character-building exercises. Each time we face a difficult situation, we get to test out our character. This really helps us to frame the situation as something that can benefit us. The setback becomes an opportunity for us to put our philosophy to the test and see what's working (and what's not working). Seneca puts it well:

"Difficulties strengthen the mind, as labour does the body."

Seneca

The more we think of things like this, the more confident we become at handling setbacks. As our confidence builds, we get better at trusting ourselves to handle whatever life throws at us. We learn to enjoy the challenge of a setback as a way for us to test out our mindsets. Very *amor fati*, you might say.

All of this is a lot easier to say than to do, so I think it's important to try this out when things don't go to plan. A good way to cultivate this attitude generally is to apply the "everything's a challenge" concept to every minor inconvenience. If there's something that you don't want to do, turn it into a character-building exercise. You can't be bothered to wash-up ... Perfect! Turn it into a challenge. Use it as an opportunity to work on your mindset. I know this isn't a setback as such, but if it's something that you don't want to do, you can still reframe the situation to turn it into something philosophical. By looking at your internal dialogue while washing up and paying attention to your thought patterns, you can turn a simple act into an opportunity to develop character. Push back against any negativity that crops up and use the mundane as a challenge.

We can also apply this idea to bigger and more demanding problems. Imagine that you've just been made redundant from your job. It was nothing personal, just a series of essential cutbacks to keep the business in profit. It would be easy to take this personally and to see this as an absolute disaster. However, reframing the situation and working with the cards you've been dealt can be liberating. The situation might actually have some silver linings ... Maybe it's the nudge you've always needed to actually leave your job and find more fulfilling work ... Maybe it's given you the chance to re-evaluate your time and your priorities ... Maybe it's given you the space to think clearly and see what other job opportunities are out there ...

If we treat every setback and inconvenience as a challenge, we can reframe it in a constructive way. We can essentially learn to think of tricky situations as a way to build resilience. This is a wonderful approach to have to setbacks!

The Stoics believed that any obstacle could be turned into an opportunity. One of Aurelius' most popular quotes is all about this:

"The impediment to action advances action.
What stands in the way becomes the way."
Marcus Aurelius

What I believe he means by this is that even when we face obstacles, we can use them to our advantage. Interestingly, the incredibly popular book *The Obstacle is The Way* by Ryan Holiday is based on this Aurelius quote. The book focuses on turning "Trials into Triumphs" and is heavily influenced by Stoic philosophy. It looks in great depth at many people who have flipped negatives into positives throughout history. You should definitely add it to your reading list.

By seeing obstacles as opportunities, we can completely change the way we feel about them. I think that one of the most effective ways to do this is to look for the lesson. When facing a big challenge, looking for something concrete and helpful to take away from the experience means that we give value to everything that happens to us. Even massive failures and problems along the way suddenly have immense value as we know that we will be able to extract lessons from them.

KINTSUGI

In Japan there's a lovely art form called *kintsugi*. When something like a plate or a piece of pottery breaks, the repairer glues it back together with golden glue. They don't try to disguise the break, but they highlight it with gold. The cracks become a part of the object and make it even more beautiful. Every plate, bowl, vase or cup that's had the *kintsugi* treatment is unique. The faults and imperfections are celebrated. In England if something breaks, it gets thrown out or recycled! Once it's broken, that's it. Goodbye! Sayonara! Personally, I like the idea of golden repair work.

I believe that we can take this further and apply the concept of *kintsugi* to our lives. Rather than try to hide our faults, imperfections and traumas, we should embrace them as part of who we are. Setbacks and difficulties can help to define us. So, we should be proud of our scars! They might have been tough to deal with at the time, but I think it's important that we learn to accept them and allow them to be part of us. We are all the more beautiful because of what we have been through. Yes, even the tough stuff.

FINAL THOUGHTS

Setbacks can teach us so much about ourselves. One of my greatest setbacks was having to learn to deal with anxiety, but in hindsight this has been one of the best things that has happened to me – it's taught me so much about who I am and led me to discover Stoicism. And to start writing books! What we can initially perceive to be devastating can, in time, turn into a profoundly transformative experience.

So, the next time you face a challenge or difficult setback, try to frame it as an opportunity – an opportunity to test your ability to handle difficulty and an opportunity to turn an obstacle into something great. And while you're at it, keep Epictetus' words close to hand:

*"For every challenge, remember the resources
you have within you to cope with it."*

Epictetus

PRACTICAL EXERCISES

The purpose of the following exercises is to get better at dealing with setbacks.

THE CONTROL LIST

The next time you face a difficult situation or setback, write a list of all the things that are within your control and all of the things that aren't. Now create a plan based solely on the things that are within your control. Focus your attention on these things and write about your experience in your journal. Did this help?

LOOK FOR THE LESSON

When things don't go to plan, look for the lesson. Try to figure out what you can learn from the experience. Make notes and then try to apply this lesson to your life going forward.

SETBACK MINDSETS

Reframe the next setback you face with one of the following mindsets:

- *The Comedy Mindset* – Look for the humour in the situation.
- *The Hero Mindset* – View yourself as the hero in a novel/ movie.
- *The Writer Mindset* – Look for content and anecdotes for your article.
- *The Stoic Mindset* – Try to be as Stoic as possible.
- *The Creative Mindset* – Look for creative solutions to the problem you are facing.

Make notes in your journal and play around with all of these mindsets. Which works best for you? Remember that it might change depending upon the setback you are dealing with.

THE SETBACK DIARY

At the end of each day create a list of setbacks that you've had to deal with and write about the solutions you came up with. They don't have to be big dramas or obstacles, although they can be if you've had to face big problems. Try to grade your performance. How did you handle the setback? Did it go well? What would you give yourself out of 10? By the way, 10 represents handling the setback like a pro without any complaints.

EVERYTHING'S A CHALLENGE

For this exercise, you need to view every frustrating situation as a test of character. Try turning the minutia of the day into character-building challenges – washing up/taking the bins out/grocery shopping, etc. Inject play into the mundane and build character while doing boring things.

JOURNALING PROMPTS

When journaling on this Stoic idea, I think that The Setback Diary is a good place to start. It helps you to think about all of the setbacks and your solutions in a structured way. Actively grading your performance is also a fantastic means to monitor progress. If you adopt this exercise on a regular basis, you will be able to observe if you are getting better at handling setbacks over time.

Creating your control list is also another great way of hashing out solutions to problems. Write down everything that you can and can't control and fill your journal with The Stoic Golden Rule in action.

6

PRINCIPLE 4: SELF-REFLECTION

"If a person doesn't know to which port they sail, no wind is favourable."

Seneca

SUMMARY OF PRINCIPLE

Wisdom and self-reflection help us to live better lives.

PRINCIPLE

The Stoics are big fans of self-reflection and encourage us to regularly spend time contemplating our actions. The way we conduct ourselves is important in Stoic philosophy as there's a heavy emphasis on ethics and personal behaviour. As mentioned earlier in the book, developing a good and virtuous character is seen as an integral part of the philosophy and one of its most important goals. Arguably, it's the most important goal, and a key way to work toward this is through self-reflection.

The Stoics saw self-reflection as an essential daily practice. Seneca made time in the morning and evening to reflect and study; Aurelius found downtime to write *Meditations* (essentially a self-reflective journal) and many modern Stoics incorporate self-reflection into their daily routine.

Self-reflection from a Stoic perspective is the ability to look at how we are living our lives and make sure that our actions align with our values. This sounds great on paper, but one question naturally crops up ... Where should we be getting these values from? We can't just open a fortune cookie and find our values.

For the Stoics, deciding how to live a good life came from wisdom. This is one of The Cardinal Virtues and is hugely important when it comes to self-reflection. So, where do we find this wisdom? Well, the Stoics would suggest philosophy as our first port of call. In fact, the Stoics would say that philosophy holds the answers to all of our problems.

Essentially, there are two aspects to this Stoic principle. The first being to study wisdom – to search for ideas and values that can guide us in life. And the second being to self-reflect on our actions to ensure that we are aligned with those ideas and values.

> *"Nobody can lead a happy life or even a bearable one without the pursuit of wisdom."*
>
> Seneca

KNOW THYSELF

Personally, I think that wisdom can come from many different places. As long as I'm seeking it out, I'm not so worried about where it comes from. For me, it's likely to be a mix of direct experience and various sources like books, teachers, mentors, role models and the Internet (although I pay close attention to how credible my online sources are – cat memes might be hilarious but they aren't the best source of life advice).

I'm always open to new concepts and am inspired by a variety of different subjects. Some of my favourite ideas come from philosophy, science, biographies and modern psychology. But many other areas inspire me deeply. Seeking out wisdom from a cross-section of sources has allowed me to self-reflect in a meaningful way. I love finding new ideas that help me to live a better life.

Socrates is famous for the saying "Know thyself", and I feel that this advice is fundamental to self-reflection. The Stoics loved Socrates, so the idea of introspection became an important part of Stoicism. Getting to know ourselves is so important. Even if we think that we know who we are, there is always more to learn.

Personality tests are a wonderful way to start the ball rolling with all of this. They can also be a lot of fun. My absolute favourite being the Myers-Briggs Type Indicator. I remember reading out this personality assessment for my friend Matt on a climbing trip and it was so accurate that we were both roaring with laughter. It's like someone knew him personally! The test was also spot on for me – (I'm an INFP in case you were wondering – Introvert/Intuition/Feeling/Perceiving).

There are a bazillion personality tests out there but for me the Myers-Briggs Type Indicator is great for drilling down into personal values. It's an interesting system, and although not part of Stoicism, it can be a helpful tool when self-reflecting and looking at personal behaviour.

Another component of getting to know yourself better and cultivating wisdom is reading. I also feel that reading broadly and diversely has helped me gain a better understanding of my values and establish how I want to live my life.

I recommend becoming your own book doctor …. Whenever you face a problem in life, look for a book that might help. For example: if you're struggling with a relationship, read a book on relationships. If you're starting a business, read a book on starting a business. If you're learning Mongolian throat singing, read a book about Mongolian throat singing. This is a practical and incredibly effective way of managing problems and exploring the specific situations you face in life.

You could take this idea further to help those around you. When your friend complains about having too much on, you can recommend *Essentialism* by Greg McKeown. For someone about to become a parent, you could gift them *The Book You Wish Your Parents Had Read* by Philippa Perry. When someone is experiencing bad anxiety, tell them about *The Chimp Paradox* by Steve Peters. The more books you read, the better you get at doing this (any excuse to buy more books, right). It can be rewarding giving book recommendations to friends and family in times of need, so why not give it a try?

When you've brushed up on your wisdom and have a better sense of the values and ideas that are important to you, it's time to reflect on your current actions and see if they are aligned. This is where self-reflection begins.

JOURNALING

The most obvious place to start when discussing the actual self-reflection process is journaling. This was a tool the ancient Stoics used to explore their thoughts on the page. *Meditations* by Aurelius, one of the most important philosophy books of all time, was never meant for publication. It was essentially his diary. So yes, we're all being nosey by reading it and constantly quoting it. Imagine writing a diary and then, 2,000 years later, extracts from it were all over the Internet! It's incredible how relatable Aurelius' words are but this was his humble way of engaging in self-reflection and making sure that he was living in alignment with his philosophy. It wasn't written for anyone else – just remember that the next time you read an Aurelius quote!

Keeping a diary can be cathartic. There's something powerful about putting pen to paper and we can see many examples of journaling as a way of managing difficult situations throughout history. One of the most moving examples being the diary of Anne Frank. I'm sure you know her story and might have even read her diary. During the Second World War, Anne and her family had to go into hiding (they were a Jewish family living in Amsterdam and were being persecuted by the Nazis).

The Franks ended up living in a secret annex above Anne's father's place of work for two years before being caught. Anne was 13 years old when they first went into hiding and during this time, she wrote a diary. This was her creative way to process what she was going through.

Anne's diary is incredibly important – not just for her, but for all of us. It's a very moving read and allows countless people access to a deeper understanding of those dark days. By hearing her story, we are reminded how we must never let anything like this happen again. Her diary has had a global impact and influenced a vast amount of people. All of this come from her finding the time to sit down and emotionally open up on the page.

There are many ways that you can use a journal in your life so it's important to find out what works best for you. Testing out a few different methods is a good place to start. This is why I've been encouraging you to journal while working through this book. Each principle has journaling prompts and is tied in with the Stoic idea of self-reflection. It's a transformative tool, so I encourage you to keep going with it.

Personally, I use a journal as a way to reflect on the day and remember key events. I also find that it helps me to be clear with my thinking, goals and ideas. I've included an entry from my journal to give you an example of how I structure my writing. You can use this as inspiration for what to do or what not to do. I've gone with a "normal day" rather than a crazy day packed with adventure.

Monday 12 July, 2021

Overview:
Woke up early – slept well. Quick walk with Helen before head down to write. Mainly a writing day. 10k run after lunch. Zoom call with client about speaking engagement. Evening meditation was good today (20 mins). Watched some stand-up comedy before bed with Hels.

Highlights:
Connected with nature on run.
Pizza with Helen.
Random nice message on Instagram from stranger.

Lessons:
Distracted on walk – be more present. Leave phone at home or turn on to silent.
Watch more comedy!

Tomorrow's important goals:
Finish self-reflection principle and reread all edits from today.
Test mic for podcast on the 15th – make sure to find and charge headphones in advance.

It doesn't take much time for me to write my journal each day so it's pretty easy to keep the habit up. Knowing that I'll be done in a few minutes helps me to commit to the process of self-reflection. It's a relatively small act but it's worth it.

The other great thing about journaling is you start to spot themes and patterns that aren't always obvious. Every couple of months I will read back over what I've written and it can provide real insight. When you keep failing to take on board a particular lesson, spotting it as a recurring pattern is incredibly helpful.

THE MORNING ROUTINE

Ah – the morning routine. You can't beat it! This is something that has been a wonderful addition to my life. Creating structure in the morning is one of the most important habits that I've introduced to my day. The thing is, this idea isn't new. Having a structure for the start of the day is old wisdom. It's been around for yonks. Personally, I like Aurelius' advice for the morning:

> *"When you arise in the morning, think of what a precious privilege it is to be alive – to breathe, to think, to enjoy, to love."*
>
> Marcus Aurelius

By starting the day reflecting on the things we are grateful for, it can help to put us in a positive frame of mind. Not a bad way to start the day.

Seneca had a slight twist on this and suggested preparation for the day ahead with some negative visualization (see Principle 6).

> *"The wise will start each day with the thought, 'Fortune gives us nothing which we can really own.' Nothing, whether public or private, is stable."*
>
> Seneca

By being conscious of the impermanence of everything, especially the things we encounter during the day, we increase our gratitude for them. Knowing that these could be taken away from us at any moment and that our lives could change in a finger snap, we start the day from a place of appreciation.

The Stoic advice is to spend some time reflecting on the day ahead when we first wake up. Creating a little routine or habit for this is a great way to put this practice into action.

A little morning routine is the perfect time for self-reflection – reading a book (preferably something packed with wisdom), spending time quietly contemplating the day ahead, meditating, engaging your body with exercise or doing an energetic crazy dance – anything goes! The thing to remember is that this time should be for you. This is where YOU carve out space in the day to think, to reflect and to ponder the wonders of life.

If you don't give yourself a moment to prepare for the day, it's easy to feel like you are being dragged through it. The days where I don't work through my morning routine are often the days where I feel as if I'm tied to a long rope with an angry rhinoceros on the other end … and it's running away from me!

Starting the day off well has a huge impact on the rest of the day. Typically, my morning routine looks something like the following:

1. Wake up (usually pretty early)
2. Stoic maxims/Negative Visualization/*memento mori* – I explain these later in the book
3. Exercise
4. Cold shower
5. Meditate
6. Read

Nothing fancy. Nothing too crazy. It usually takes between an hour to two hours to work through everything – but they can be condensed if needed. My routine does change depending upon where I am, but these are the things that help to set me up for the day ahead. If I can tick all of these off my list, I know that I have set myself up for a good day.

When creating your own routine, think about what would suit your lifestyle. For Seneca it usually started with some exercise, followed by cold-water bathing and then some simple food. For you, it might be naked press-ups followed by Marmite on toast ... There are so many options to try. Journaling a little on what your morning routine could look like will be time well spent.

THE EVENING ROUTINE

The end of the day provides us with the perfect opportunity to really put all of this self-reflection into action. Looking back over the day is a highly effective way of ensuring that we are truly living in alignment with our values. Was it really necessary to shout at that dog? Did you have to swear so much when you dropped your toast? Why didn't you hold the door for that person? Exactly! Now, go to your room and think about what you've done!

Epictetus encourages us to reflect on the day in a specific way:

*"Allow not sleep to lose your wearied eyes,
until you have reckoned up each daytime
deed: Where did I go wrong? What did I do?
And what duty's left undone? From first to last
review your acts and then reprove yourself
for wretched (or cowardly) acts, but rejoice in
those done well."*

Epictetus

The beauty of looking back over the day in the evening is that everything is fresh in our minds. Well, as fresh as it's ever going to be. We should be able to run through what's happened in the day and draw a line under it without having to scratch our heads too much. The important thing to remember when doing this is that making mistakes throughout the day is natural. We need to accept what didn't go well and not beat ourselves up if things didn't go to plan. As long as we look for the lesson and don't dwell on the negative, we will be self-reflecting in a way that helps us to stay positive and keep on track!

Assigning time at the end of the day to think about our actions can be a transformative exercise. It's a very Stoic thing to do.

FINAL THOUGHTS

Carving out time in the day to both cultivate wisdom and self-reflect on our behaviour is a very important habit. In reality, it doesn't have to be a huge chunk of time … I feel that consistency is more important than length of time spent doing it. A few minutes at each end of the day will work well. In the morning, a little routine where we reflect on the day ahead and prepare in a way that suits us is a great place to start. In the evening, a short look over the events of the day and how we behaved can be highly effective. Making a few notes in a journal along the way can help ensure that we are living in alignment with our values and that we are self-reflecting Stoically.

"I will keep constant watch over myself and – most usefully – will put each day up for review. For this is what makes us evil – that none of us looks back upon our own lives. We reflect upon only that which we are about to do. And yet

our plans for the future descend
from the past."
Seneca

PRACTICAL EXERCISES

The purpose of these exercises is to help increase self-awareness and establish time for self-reflection.

MORNING ROUTINE

Start your day off the right way by working through a morning routine. Create your own and test it out for a month. Start with something not too demanding and add to it over time. Things like exercise, meditation and reading work well and are great ways to start the day. But the ball is in your court here, so go for a routine and activities that work for you.

EVENING ROUTINE

In the style of the Stoics, end your day with a little self-reflection. This might be some quiet time spent reviewing the day or actively journaling. In fact, journaling and the evening routine complement each other really well. Like a mouse with cheese, they were destined to be together. So why not try to include a little writing time in your evening routine?

Here's a great structure inspired by Epictetus for you to try. By running through three simple questions, we are extracting the most value from the day:

What didn't go to plan today? Looking at what went wrong helps us to learn from our mistakes. It's also an opportunity to check if we responded to situations healthily – did we get into a flap and lose control of our minds? Or did we handle the obstacles gracefully?

What went well today? Looking at what went well has useful lessons too – it can teach us what works and how to go about making that happen again. It's also an opportunity to focus on what we are thankful for and to cultivate more gratitude for everything positive that occurred throughout the day.

What needs to be done tomorrow? Looking at what is coming up allows us to plan ahead and be prepared for what's around the corner. Handy, if you've got a lot on your plate.

Try creating an evening routine that helps you to successfully close the day. Now implement it for a month.

THE BOOK DOCTOR

Become your own book doctor. In this exercise, you need to select a problem you are facing in life right now and then read a book about it. The problem can be anything – health-related, about a relationship or career problems. Literally anything. Your chosen book will (hopefully) give you the wisdom to move forward with your problem.

This exercise can be expanded further by creating a comprehensive list of your life problems and a book bucket-list to help you address those issues.

JOURNALING

Spend a week reflectively journaling on your day. Ask yourself what went well and what didn't. Look at your behaviour, why you acted the way you did, and consider how you could have improved the day.

KNOW THYSELF

Spend some time getting to know yourself better. Try a few personality tests to gain some wisdom and insight into your behaviour. I recommend the Myers-Briggs Type Indicator. You might also want to check out the DISC method.

JOURNALING PROMPTS

For this principle, I suggest that you follow the evening routine exercise and spend time reflectively looking through your day. There are multiple ways to do this but, as mentioned earlier, looking for lessons and highlights can work well. This means that the focus is on improvement rather than things that you did badly.

7

PRINCIPLE 5: ROLE MODELS

"For we must indeed have someone according to whom we may regulate our characters; you can never straighten that which is crooked unless you use a ruler."

Seneca

SUMMARY OF PRINCIPLE

Role models can guide us by showing us how to behave in the world.

PRINCIPLE

I really love the Seneca quote from the start of this principle. It's one of my all-time favourite Stoic quotes and does a wonderful job of highlighting the importance of role models in our lives. Without good role models, it's hard to cultivate the right attitude toward life.

As Stoic philosophy encourages us to develop virtuous characters, emulating the behaviour of those who live "virtuous" lives makes total sense. When someone exemplifies good behaviour, that should be seen as a benchmark for how we should behave. If someone does something kind and admirable, we can use this as inspiration.

Role models come in a variety of different forms and the Stoics had a bunch of them. Cato, Plato and Diogenes were pretty popular. Epicurus the philosopher was one of Seneca's favourites (even though he wasn't a Stoic). Many of the Roman Stoics also looked back at the former heads of the Stoic school – Zeno, Cleanthes and Chrysippus. These philosophers and their behaviour would be seen as inspiring figures.

Aurelius kicks off his timeless *Meditations* with a long list of people who have inspired him in life. He systematically goes through family members, teachers and friends and writes down what important life lesson he's taken from them. Role models galore!

Socrates was also frequently referenced by the Stoics and seen as a hugely important figure. Although not a Stoic, his life and ideas were influential to them. Epictetus gives us a hint at how highly they regarded him with the following quote:

"... Socrates fulfilled himself by attending to nothing except reason in everything that he encountered. And you, although you are not yet a Socrates, should live as someone who at least wants to be a Socrates."

Epictetus

According to Epictetus, we should aspire to live like Socrates, and use his behaviour as a benchmark for what to do and how to live a good life.

The reality is, we can pick and choose our role models and they don't have to be from philosophy. They can come from a diverse range of sources. But, how do we find them?

HOW TO PICK ROLE MODELS

Role models can come from all over the place – family members, friends, colleagues, inspirational figures in society, teachers, writers ... The list will likely be different for all of us. My role models won't be the same as yours. And vice versa.

When selecting role models, the Stoic solution would be to look for those with good character: people who make the world a better place, who inspire us to be kinder and the best we can possibly be.

So, what is "good character"? According to the Stoics, this is found in someone who lives a virtuous life. It is someone who follows The Cardinal Virtues (Wisdom, Justice, Fortitude, Temperance) and lives within a strong ethical framework – someone who acts with the right intentions and works hard to be a decent human being. This is how the Stoics would judge someone and decide if they made the cut for their role models list.

We don't necessarily have to use these parameters, and we will all judge what we would consider to be a good character slightly differently (and this might even change over time). Personal values like kindness, honesty and empathy are all on my list when I think of "good character" and look for role models. What about you?

Spend a bit of time thinking about who would make the cut for your list and then start creating it. This can be a fun process. When adding someone, ask yourself what qualities and characteristics have made you add them to the list.

My list is pretty long. A lot of my role models are close friends and family, and many come from biographies I've read. Interestingly, a lot of them aren't even alive. It's a real cross-section! One of the most important role models in my life is Helen. My wife is a real Stoic about so many things and inspires me infinitely. I'm so incredibly lucky to have her in my life. I hope you have a Helen in your life.

So, what happens next? Well, when we've selected a bunch of these people we admire, we can then use their behaviour and actions as inspiration.

It's worth mentioning at this point that we do need to be careful when comparing ourselves to others ...

Nowadays, we tend to spend a lot of time comparing ourselves to other people. I mean, I'm sure we used to do this in the past – "Why is Fred's cave bigger than mine? And look at his woolly mammoth jacket ... I can't believe he's got that. I want one!" But in modern life, social media allows us so much access to other people's "supposed" daily lives. Naturally, we can't help but make comparisons ... When we follow our favourite celebrities or successful people on social media, we get an insight into a life that might look very different to our own.

This type of comparison isn't ideal as it often tends to come from a place of envy and jealousy. The type of comparison that is more in alignment with Stoicism is a comparison of character. What type of person are they? It's not the lifestyle that's important, it's their character. And if they have a good character, its nothing to be jealous of, but something to aspire to!

ANTI-ROLE MODELS

What's the opposite of a role model? An anti-role model! These are the people whose behaviour we don't want to emulate. The truth is, we won't have to look far to find these people. Bad behaviour is out there. This is the way the world works – whether we like it or not.

I'm sure you can think of many people who would fill the anti-role model shoes (I can think of plenty). They might be people we personally know, they might be random people we encounter out and about or they might be in the media spotlight. It probably won't take long for you to create a list of these people. In fact, I'd encourage you to start thinking about these people now. What is it about them that you dislike? What qualities and characteristics do they possess that you think are less than desirable?

This might initially seem like quite a negative exercise, but it isn't at all. We are looking at behaviour that we don't want to copy and observing it in others. We are looking for negative characteristics and using that as an example of what we shouldn't do. Sometimes, knowing what not to do can be incredibly helpful.

Our anti-role models don't just have to be dictators, serial killers and corrupt politicians. We can also find small examples of poor behaviour and use that as a guide for what we should avoid doing. For example, if someone cuts us up in traffic, we can use them as an anti-role model. Rather than get angry at them, we should try to do the exact opposite of what they are doing and make a conscious effort to never cut others up when driving. Granted, they might not be a full-blown anti-role model, but we can use their negative characteristics as something we aim to avoid.

The anti-role model gets us thinking about the negative traits that we might possess and encourages us to consciously take action against them. This idea forces us to look at our own behaviour and make sure that it isn't aligned with our anti-role models' behaviour.

I think Aurelius summed all of this up perfectly:

"The best revenge is not to be like your enemy."

Aurelius

THE STOIC SAGE

We have superheroes. I mean, we don't really have them – but they exist as a concept. These fictional characters have incredible powers that allow them to do superhuman things: Spiderman (my personal favourite), Wonder Woman, Batman, Cat Woman, Black Panther, The Avengers, etc. Often, you'll find them fighting evil and saving the world. Granted, a lot of them have their own "issues" that they're dealing with but they typically illustrate good and virtuous behaviour. When we're younger, superheroes can teach us a lot about morals and ethics and inspire us to be good people. Interestingly, it's not just younger generations that these superheroes inspire – people of all ages flock to see the latest superhero movie. The triumph of good over evil is a timeless narrative that appeals to many.

The Stoics actually had their own imaginary superhero – the Stoic Sage (who did not wield a lightsabre, sadly). The Stoic Sage is a hypothetical person who lives the perfect philosophical life. Whatever happens to them, they handle it perfectly. Their behaviour and character are faultless. Obviously, that's pretty much impossible. No one is perfect and the greatest people to have walked this planet had faults. We know that perfection doesn't exist, but that doesn't mean we can't contemplate what that might look like. Thus, the hypothetical Stoic Sage appears.

By thinking about what the Sage would do when facing a problem, we get a clear representation of what Stoicism in action looks like. It's all very well spending years studying philosophical concepts but if we don't map this onto our behaviour, it can seem like a waste of time. Picturing what this would look like on someone is helpful.

The Stoic Sage is essentially all of the ideas from Stoicism compressed into a human form. The Sage represents how we should strive to act in each moment. I wrote about the idea of *aretê* at the start of the book – being the best possible version of ourselves in every instance. Well, the Stoic Sage is the perfect manifestation of that. Ideally, we should aim to try to act like that Sage at all times.

WHAT WOULD THE STOICS DO?

The Stoics are fantastic role models for all of us in terms of self-control, the ability to think clearly and choosing our response to situations – all practices that are helpful for us.

When we find ourselves in a tricky situation and aren't sure about the best course of action, we should ask the question: "What would the Stoics do?" Thinking about how they would handle everything can lead to practical solutions to large and small problems.

Personally, I like the idea of receiving an imaginary pep talk from one of the ancient Stoics. In my first book I wrote about Epictetus giving a motivating speech after you hypothetically break your leg. It was quite silly but I think his advice was sound. It mainly focused on what you can and can't control (but that's to be expected from Epictetus).

Visualizing your favourite Stoic role model coming and yakking away about your problem can be a fun exercise. You might even write to yourself in the style of one of the Stoics. Seneca used to write letters to Lucilius about many different issues. Just pretend that you're Seneca writing to yourself. This gets you into the Stoic headspace and can be an effective way to synthesize all of this Stoic philosophy you've been reading about. It also helps you to view your problem objectively which can give you some distance from it.

You can take all of this further by contemplating the Stoic Sage. As mentioned before, this theoretical person exemplifies "perfect" behaviour. They are the ultimate role model ... Whatever happens to them, they handle it like a pro. So, imagine them in a pickle, and then what they would do to get out of said pickle. When you've figured it out, do that!

YOU ARE A ROLE MODEL

It's easy to forget the influence we have on others. Whether we are aware of it or not, people look at us and judge our behaviour. It might not always be a conscious process, but people do. Without fail.

Our perception of how we think others see us can dramatically alter our behaviour and make us feel self-conscious. We worry about how those around us view our actions, and about being judged by them. But this is part of life. Everything we do is judged. Every move we make. Every step we take. They'll be watching us. That was what Sting said, right?

Knowing that we are being watched by those around us should inspire us to behave well. Our actions can determine whether we are anti-role models or role models to others so think carefully about how you live your life.

It's worth noting that impressionable people might struggle to differentiate good from bad behaviour. This is particularly true for children and young people. If you have someone little in your life, they don't understand what an anti-role model is. You are just a role model, so your behaviour will be copied. Remember that the next time you're about to do something stupid.

Becoming conscious of what type of role model you are to others is a helpful exercise. Think about all of the people in your life. What do you think they think about you? Have you ever stopped to ponder this? What characteristics would they say you had? Why not write down a list of these characteristics and then actually ask the people in your life to tell you how they see you? The truth could be very different to what you think. Compare lists and see what you got right/wrong.

Think about the fact that people are watching you. How do you want them to remember you? What do you want them to say? When you've worked this out, start acting appropriately.

FINAL THOUGHTS

Role models can play an important part in our self-development. The goal of contemplating these role models (both positive and negative) is to make us more aware of these people in our lives. When we have more awareness of their behaviour, we can make sure that we are either emulating good behaviour or avoiding bad behaviour. It sounds pretty obvious but there's something powerful about experiencing this process first-hand. When we are inspired by someone's actions or ideas, it motivates us to make important changes in our lives.

"Take a good hard look at people's ruling principle, especially of the wise, what they run away from and what they seek out."

Marcus Aurelius

PRACTICAL EXERCISES

The purpose of these exercises is to give guidance on how to live by following the examples of others.

ROLE MODELS
The goal of this specific exercise is to establish your role models and use their behaviour as a benchmark. This can be from a wide range of sources – family/friends/people you admire/ athletes/writers/philosophers/Stoics, etc.

List these people in your journal or on a digital device and write down the qualities that you admire in them. Study your role models and collect quotes and coping mechanisms from them. Now think about ways you might emulate their behaviour and characteristics in your life.

ANTI-ROLE MODELS

Spend some time collecting examples of anti-role models and list the qualities that you want to avoid in your life. Now avoid behaving like this at all costs!

A little side note – You might not want to announce your anti-role models publicly, so it's probably best to keep your list private.

THE STOIC SAGE

Create a list of virtues that you think a Stoic Sage would have. Now contemplate what the perfect reaction to difficult situations would look like. How would the Stoic Sage deal with the following:

- Someone being rude
- A small obstacle
- A large obstacle
- Bad news
- Good news
- Personal injury

Create a list of more problems and think about what the perfect solution would look like.

YOU ARE A ROLE MODEL

Spend time thinking about the people who would consider you a role model – Children? Friends? Colleagues? Family members? Strangers? Are you being the best version of yourself for the people who need you in their lives? Focus on being that role model – what would the best possible version of yourself be/look like? This will link back to *aretê* and The Cardinal Virtues mentioned at the start of the book.

Why not test all of this out by writing a list of how you think others see you and then compare notes with what they actually say?

WHAT WOULD THE STOICS DO?

When facing a problem in life, think about how the Stoics would deal with it. By asking yourself what Aurelius/Epictetus/Seneca would do in this situation, you have a framework for how to handle that problem.

You can take all of this further by mapping different role models' responses onto your problem (not just the Stoics). Who has the best solution?

JOURNALING PROMPTS

For this principle the main goal is to build up your list of role models and anti-role models. After you have established this, reflect on the type of qualities you want to bring into your life. Explore what characteristics are desirable and look for recurring themes in your role model choice. How can you disrupt this? Are there those who break the theme but would also be great role models? Look for different types of role models and seek out people that you don't know about.

You can also use your journal as a way to reflect on the people you encounter out and about. Note if they would fall into a role model or anti-role model camp. It's interesting to think that some people might actually have qualities that fall into both camps. Pick the qualities you admire and try to explore and incorporate them in your daily life.

8

PRINCIPLE 6: NEGATIVE VISUALIZATION

"Rehearse them in your mind: exile, torture, war, shipwreck. All the terms of our human lot should be before our eyes."

Seneca

WARNING

This is an advanced Stoic concept. It can be extremely difficult for some people to use and, if done incorrectly, it can put you in a very negative mental space. Be particularly careful if you are experiencing anxiety, depression or any other mental health conditions. Feel free to skip the principle if it's too much. You can always come back to it at a later stage.

SUMMARY OF PRINCIPLE

Think about what could go wrong so that it doesn't catch you off guard. This idea can also be used to heighten your sense of gratitude for everything in life.

PRINCIPLE

Most of us are familiar with positive visualization – by thinking about positive outcomes, we help our brains to focus on achieving these things. Competitive athletes are encouraged to visualize themselves standing on the podium with a gold medal and cheering crowds. We're told to picture the job interview going well and all of the wonderful things that will happen afterwards. This idea can be used for a whole host of situations and lots of people have had great success with positive visualization. However, the Stoics had a slightly different approach. They actively explored the opposite – negative visualization. This is essentially imagining negative things and situations in great detail.

Negative visualization can be used for two main purposes:

1. To anticipate future problems so that you are better prepared to face them.
2. To create a heightened appreciation for life itself and a deep sense of gratitude for everything.

The first reason – to be prepared for what might go wrong – is something that we see in the modern world all the time. The concept makes total sense. If a new business is launching, it would be reckless not to think about how it might fail. The business founder/s will likely use a SWOT analysis, where they systematically explore the strengths, weaknesses, opportunities and threats that the business might face. This is common practice for new businesses and projects. Imagine opening a giant techno super-club in a town where the population was mainly older folks ... No one would turn up!

If we don't anticipate things that might not work or things that could go wrong, we are in danger of being caught off guard. Being aware of threats can help us to prepare. I'm pretty confident that you don't spend all day thinking about a fire in your home, but by spending a little time doing a risk assessment, you would likely agree that a fire alarm and a fire extinguisher are good investments. This is why I have both of these in my home. I hope to never use the fire extinguisher, but if there is a fire, I have a handy way of dealing with it. This is not paranoia; it's preparing for a potential worst-case scenario.

This all sounds very "health and safety" and I guess in a way it is. But the Stoics weren't going around with clipboards stopping people from having fun. They were just conscious of what might go wrong. Epictetus said:

> *"When you are going to perform an act, remind yourself what kind of things the act may involve. When going to the swimming pool, reflect on what may happen at the pool: some will splash the water, some will push against one another, others will abuse one another, and others will steal. Thusly you have mentally prepared yourself to undertake the act, and you can say to yourself: I now intend to bathe, and am prepared to maintain my will in a virtuous manner, having warned myself of what may occur."*
>
> Epictetus

I don't know about you, but this doesn't sound like the kind of pool I'd fancy going to on a Sunday morning. But we can see how Epictetus' thinking would help him to not get worked up if some random bloke tried to steal his stuff and splash him with water ...

Seneca mirrors this sentiment when he talked about us having unrealistic expectations of reality. If we think that we live in a world where things don't go wrong, or bad stuff never happens, we are going to be constantly disappointed. It's on us to learn that reality is a mixed bag of events. Sometimes good stuff happens; sometimes bad stuff happens. What's important is how we deal with it. And the Stoics believed that a great way to deal with bad stuff happening is to have spent some time in advance thinking about these things and creating a plan.

NEGATIVE VISUALIZATION IN THE MODERN WORLD

My favourite modern example of this is Alex Honnold. Alex is a world-renowned rock climber who featured in the Oscar-winning documentary *Free Solo*. The beautifully shot film follows Alex as he prepares and then climbs the route "Freerider" in Yosemite, USA. He does this without a rope. That's pretty much 1,000 metres of vertical granite without any protection. No rope. No gear. Just shoes and a chalk bag. Watching him climb the route is intense. It's undeniably one of the most incredible human achievements in sporting history. Just watch it and I'm sure you'll agree. Get ready for some sweaty palms ...

The thing that links Alex to the Stoics is the way he prepared for the climb. Along with using positive visualization to imagine successfully climbing the route, he also pictured what might go wrong – the perfect example of negative visualization.

Alex imagined all of the things that he could potentially encounter on the climb so that he would mentally know how to deal with them if they were to actually happen. There were heaps of variables to consider – what would happen if a bird flew out of one of the cracks and into his face? What if he met other climbers on the route? What would he do if he wanted to retreat? What would happen if the weather suddenly changed?

What would he do if he really needed the toilet? The list could go on and on.

Alex also thought about what would happen if he were to fall … By spending time imagining a fall (essentially contemplating his own death), he mentally prepared himself for that possibility. Suddenly thinking about the consequences of a fall halfway up the climb would have been a terrible idea; his body and mind could quickly freak out under the pressure. This would then cause adrenaline to shoot through his veins and a panicking mind could make him lose control of the situation. This panic and fear could ultimately kill him. Alex needed to be in complete control for the climb to be successful and intense fear would have gotten in the way. By exploring all of the potential outcomes on the ground (especially thinking about what might go wrong), he was better equipped to climb the route, using the negatives as a way to prepare. Very Stoic.

To be fair, climbing in general is filled with risk assessments and negative visualization. I've certainly used this technique to run through what might go wrong when out in the mountains or at the local cliff/crag/boulders. Is this route safe for me to climb? Is it a good idea to wear a helmet? Is the weather too bad for me to head off into the mountains? Have I tied my knot properly? The fact that miscalculations could result in death means that thinking about what might go wrong is essential. Negative visualization is incredibly practical.

Now, by this point you're probably thinking that the Stoics were a right bunch of miserable moaners. By constantly thinking about the negative, surely, they had a pessimistic outlook on life. It's easy to think this but it's actually not the case. The Stoics viewed all of these "negatives" as "indifferences" – like the exile. The idea is that circumstances and events don't define who we are. We might not want negative things to happen, but they don't have to destroy our character if they do. To the

Stoics, negatives are just obstacles and there is nothing gloomy about having to face them.

So, that's the first way negative visualization can help us – by being prepared for what might happen. The second way is to help us increase our gratitude. By thinking about stuff going wrong or by contemplating loss, we can increase our appreciation for life as it is right now. Contemplating loss is an interesting type of negative visualization and can be particularly powerful.

CONTEMPLATING LOSS

"Remember that all we have is 'on loan' from Fortune, which can reclaim it without our permission – indeed, without even advance notice. Thus, we should love all our dear ones, but always with the thought that we have no promise that we may keep them forever – nay, no promise that we may keep them for long."

Seneca

Thinking about important things being taken from us is a great way to increase appreciation. If we never consider the importance of what we have in life, we can easily become ungrateful.

The Stoics would spend time imagining losing loved ones, friends and possessions. All of this might sound a little morbid and depressing, but it wasn't meant to be. It was there to help increase their appreciation for life.

If we are conscious of how temporary everything is, we value what we have more. Thinking about the fact that we have limited time with our friends and family helps us to appreciate the time we actually spend with them. It'll likely make us more attentive when we are in their presence and this is a great way to build deeper relationships with people. Every time we see someone, it might be the last time ... We should therefore act accordingly. We don't need to be overly dramatic about this but we should ensure that we always leave things well and that we show kindness and compassion.

It's too easy to take things for granted in life so the idea of contemplating loss is the perfect counter. Here are a few things that we can contemplate losing: partner, family, friends, pets, personal health, senses, limbs, job, money, home, car, laptop, phone, TV, clothes, sentimental objects.

The list could go on, and it will also look different for each of us. Try the exercise at the end of this principle if you feel strong enough.

IT COULD BE WORSE

Another way that the Stoics would use negative visualization would be to think about how the problems they faced could be worse. This type of Stoic thinking can be useful when dealing with an unpleasant or negative situation. Actively thinking about how much worse the situation could be brings some objectivity to it. There is ALWAYS a way something could be worse. This helps us to search for positivity in what we are actually facing.

Thinking about how the situation could be worse isn't denying what needs to be dealt with, it just helps us to see the bigger picture. Especially if we're caught up in the moment. Being catastrophic in our thinking can drag us down, so quickly running through worse-case scenarios can prompt a hint of gratitude during tough times.

As I'm writing this, my right foot is elevated on a load of cushions. My ankle is about three times the size it should be and covered in blue and yellow bruising. It looks pretty disgusting. I fell off a climb yesterday and landed awkwardly. I've had it looked at and it's a badly sprained ankle. Less than ideal, but I can still hobble around and the great news is that it isn't broken. I was obviously annoyed when this happened but I really did embrace the concept of "It could be worse." Yes, it's frustrating that I can't walk properly. Yes, it means that I can't run or hike or do any of the normal activities that I really enjoy. Yes, it's painful and makes going to the kitchen to make a cup of tea difficult (especially considering the amount of tea I drink). But … I am actually really grateful. It hasn't ruined my mood and I'm acutely aware of how much worse it could have been. I can still move around. I can still drive. I don't have to wear a boot and use crutches. I didn't have to go to the hospital. I can still write, read and meditate and do loads of the other things I love to do. It really could have been a lot worse.

I heard a great example about this type of thinking from the author and philosopher Sam Harris during an interview on his *Waking Up* app. One day a pipe burst above his living room and water started pouring through the roof. As Sam began stressing about what to do, his wife turned to him and told him to focus on the fact that at least it was only water. Imagine if it was sewage! Sam said that this brought a touch of relief to a difficult situation. They still had to deal with the problem at hand but by focusing on the fact that it wasn't sewage spewing into the living room, it helped them to find gratitude in that moment.

A lot of people do this naturally, so it's interesting to recognize it in action. When you next face a disaster, see if you can implement this type of thinking. It's a quick way to reframe a situation and can be useful for taking the sting out of something challenging.

HELLO DARKNESS, MY OLD FRIEND

There's a restaurant in London called *Dans Le Noir?* and it's unique. The whole restaurant is pitch black. You go inside, deposit your phone in a safe box (so as to not spoil the atmosphere) and your waiter leads you to a table. You are then left sitting in complete darkness. You literally can't see anything. Hold your hand an inch in front of your eyes and you still won't see it!

When I visited the restaurant, I was amazed by how heightened all of my other senses became. The noise in the restaurant seemed incredibly loud and the smells were overwhelmingly strong. It was completely disorientating and I was thrown well out of my comfort zone. Simple things like pouring my own drink instantly became difficult. Knowing where my food was also proved problematic. To add to the concoction of disorientation, I was genuinely worried that I would poke myself in the eye with the food on my fork! In all honesty, I lost my appetite.

Spending time in this restaurant gives customers an insight into what it would be like to lose their vision. This insight can be profound. The waiters at *Dans Le Noir?* are blind and navigate the darkness seamlessly. They have learned to live in complete darkness all of the time. This is their daily reality, something that can be hard for those with vision to comprehend. I have nothing but respect for those facing this challenge.

I remember walking away from the restaurant with such a deep appreciation for my sight. After two hours in complete darkness, the colours on the journey home seemed so vibrant. It was an experience I will never forget.

Unfortunately, this deep sense of gratitude can fade quickly and that's why the Stoic concept of negative visualization is so helpful to bring this idea into our lives every day.

FINAL THOUGHTS

Negative visualization is an incredibly powerful tool. Granted, it's not the easiest tool in the box to use, but if we are careful with it and don't let our thinking spiral out of control, it can enable us to appreciate what we have in life more deeply. We can use this concept to shift our perspective quickly. It's powerful, practical and humbling.

Along with a heightened sense of gratitude for what we have in our lives, negative visualization will allow us to be better prepared for misfortune. With this concept we shouldn't feel paranoid about the future, but mentally prepared for curveballs. I encourage you to test out this principle in your life. I have some specific exercises that you can try in the next section. But for now, I'll leave you with Seneca's wise words:

"Whatever has long been anticipated comes as a lighter blow."

Seneca

PRACTICAL EXERCISES

The purpose of these exercises is to increase gratitude for everything in life and to be prepared for things going wrong.

WHAT COULD POSSIBLY GO WRONG?

Think of a future task that you've got in the calendar and imagine all of the potential things that might go wrong. The task can be something simple like walking to the shops or a more important activity like a work presentation. Crack your journal out and list all the negative things that could happen.

Now come up with a solution for each of these problems in advance. Do you feel more prepared?

CONTEMPLATING LOSS

The purpose of this exercise is to cultivate a heightened sense of gratitude for everything in your life. Set a timer for five minutes and imagine how you would feel if you lost the object of your contemplation. Think about what you would do, how it would feel and how you would handle it. Make notes as soon as the timer rings and then go and spend time appreciating what you haven't actually lost.

There are three categories/scenarios to explore:

- **Easy:** Phone/Sentimental Objects/Computer/Car/Running Water/Food/Bed
- **Medium:** Home/Job/Local Area or Country (For Local Area or Country, imagine never being able to be there again)
- **Hard:** Family/Friends/Pets/Personal Health

Please note that this is a powerful exercise and, as I said earlier, contemplating loss can be very difficult. The idea is not to dwell deeply on it every second of every day (that would not be good) but to visit the thought from time to time. I've completely messed up this exercise and ended up feeling very sad on several occasions. I've done this with Helen, my family and my friends as the focal point and if I dwell on everything for too long, it's easy for the exercise to spiral out of control. This is especially true if you have a strong imagination.

I certainly wouldn't have been able to use this exercise when I was in a very anxious mind frame so I wouldn't go near this with a barge pole if you're feeling depressed, anxious, paranoid or struggling with a bad day. Make sure you are in the right mental space to do this exercise.

HELP!
What To Do if You Get Sucked into a Black Hole of Despair

OK, so you got carried away. You've let your mind snowball and now you're feeling awful and very upset.

Firstly, you need to bring yourself back into the present moment. Take a deep breath and come back to where you are right now. Look around the room you are in and notice the details – what colour are the walls? What can you see, hear and smell? Feel the seat you are sitting in or the ground beneath your feet. Wiggle your toes and stretch your body. There's a lot you can do to reconnect to the present.

Secondly, acknowledge that this is an exercise and not what is actually happening. You have got sucked into a future scenario and this is not objective reality. Focus your attention on how wonderful it is to have whatever it is you've contemplated losing in your life. Use this as a trigger to be more grateful.

Thirdly, move away from the exercise for now. You can come back to it later when you are feeling more in control and explore what happened. For now, just move away. I suggest comedy. Go and watch something funny on You-Tube. Have you seen that guy chasing his dog Fenton in Richmond Park? Well, maybe look that up. You don't have to go far to find a distraction.

Finally, when you are starting to feel a little better, have a debrief. Think about why you snowballed out of control. What happened to cause you to get sucked into the black hole?

I would recommend coming back to the exercise again but trying a lighter version. You went in too hard. Build up slowly and be careful. Visualizing things in black and white or on a small TV screen can help you to detach a little from the thoughts.

THE TOOTHBRUSH OF GRATITUDE

If directly contemplating loss is too difficult at first, this is a great stepping-stone exercise. Rather than focusing on what it would be like to not have something in your life, focus on the pure gratitude for what you do have. While brushing your teeth each night, list all of the things that you are grateful for. Maybe do it in your head to avoid spraying toothpaste all over the bathroom!

PREPPING FOR EMERGENCIES

Create a survival kit that you can use in the case of an emergency. This is a practical exercise and could end up saving your life. Think about what scenarios would warrant different kits. Head torch? First-aid kit? Water purification tablets? Survival food? Foil emergency blanket? This might sound extreme but is pretty normal practice if you live somewhere where natural disasters occur. However, it's not common practice globally. Although this is not technically a Stoic exercise, I like the way that it makes us think about what could happen and prepare accordingly. It's more of a hands-on type of negative visualization. Why not take all of this further and go on a first-aid training course? Or a self-defence course? How else can you prepare for emergencies?

IT COULD BE WORSE

When was the last time something bad happened to you? When you have this event in your mind, list ten ways that it could have been worse. The more creative, the better. By seeking out ways that it could have been worse, you bring objectivity and perspective to the situation.

To take this further, test it out in real time. When something negative happens, look for ways that it could be worse.

JOURNALING PROMPTS

The main journaling goal for this principle is to establish a deeper understanding of negative visualization and how you can effectively use it in your life. I'd recommend starting off with the practical approach of listing things that could go wrong and potential solutions. This can be helpful to feel more prepared for an event that you are particularly nervous about. Covering all eventualities enables you to draw a line under it and know that you're ready for whatever might happen.

After this, reflecting on your actual negative visualization exercises is a great use of your journaling time. It doesn't take long to jot down any thoughts and ideas that popped up and this can be helpful for cultivating gratitude.

9

PRINCIPLE 7: MANAGING STRONG EMOTIONS

"You have power over your mind – not outside events. Realize this, and you will find strength."

Marcus Aurelius

SUMMARY OF PRINCIPLE

Strong emotions can be controlled and managed with practice.

PRINCIPLE

Life can be an emotional rollercoaster. One minute you're having a great time, feeling good and enjoying your day and then suddenly something happens that flips your mood around. A negative event triggers a strong emotional response and you quickly become overwhelmed. In a matter of seconds, you lose control of the situation. Whether it's fear, anger, grief or jealousy, it doesn't normally end well.

Strong emotions can be hard to manage and are incredibly powerful forces. They can make fully grown adults behave like toddlers. Someone caught up in their emotions can do very stupid things. I'm sure you've witnessed this at some point in your life. Maybe you've been the person doing that incredibly stupid thing (don't worry, we've all been there). Out-of-control negative emotions can have serious consequences and can lead to destructive behaviour that is damaging in many ways – both internally and externally. So, learning how to manage them effectively can transform our lives. Enter the Stoics ...

The Stoics want us to have more control over our emotions. They want us to be in the driving seat and not enslaved by strong feelings. This is pretty reasonable if you ask me. Having the ability to not get overwhelmed by our emotions can help us live less reactive lives and remain level-headed when things start getting intense. All of this is very wise. But it's not always easy.

The Stoics have a specific word they use for this – *apatheia*. It's a little tricky to translate but in essence it means remaining tranquil and undisturbed by strong emotions.

A quick side note – don't get *apatheia* confused with the modern word "apathy". This sometimes happens but they are completely different words. Apathy tends to have a negative connotation and refers to a lack of feeling or concern toward something. *Apatheia*, on the other hand, is the ability to remain in control when strong emotions come knocking. Two very different things indeed.

The aim of *apatheia* isn't to remove emotions completely and become a heartless and indifferent automaton. Stoics don't look at puppies and go – "Phfffff, I am unmoved by their cuteness." They also aren't unaffected by sad news. Stoics cry. They are normal people with normal emotions. However, Stoics seek to maintain perspective so that things don't get out of control. They don't want their emotions to completely take over.

If you were to hide in a cupboard and jump out on a Stoic, they would likely leap and yelp in shock (don't try this at home). This is a normal reaction. Again, we're not trying to control or remove this type of response. This is normal human behaviour. The Stoics actually call this reaction *propatheiai*. This is essentially your reflex and initial impression to an external event.

There's a great story about a Stoic philosopher on a boat during a crazy storm. Everyone on the boat was freaking out with fear thinking that they were about to die. The Stoic also turned pale and looked terrified but didn't complain or add additional worries to the mix. The Stoic experienced fear like everybody else but didn't take it one step further and lose mental control of the situation. The story illustrates that even Stoics experience strong emotions. These initial reactions are things that we can't control in life. It's an innate response. However, we can choose how we react after the initial moment.

Another quick side note before we move on – emotions are often referred to as "Passions" by the Stoics. The word is technically a little different but you can comfortably use "emotion" and everything will still make sense. It's worth knowing this as it does come up a lot when you read the Stoics.

HOW TO DEVELOP *APATHEIA*

The Stoics have some great strategies to develop a less reactive attitude and manage our *passions*. These range from delaying our responses to situations to leaning into virtue and philosophy. Some of these ideas might be thousands of years old but they still work wonders in the modern world.

When dealing with strong emotions, the Stoics don't encourage us to repress them. This is another common misperception about Stoicism. Repressing emotions is not a good idea. Modern psychology suggests that repression is a terrible tactic and can cause more problems to crop up in different places as a result of ignoring our feelings. If you suppress your anger, you might suddenly find yourself punching a loaf of bread later in the day. OK, that might seem a ridiculous example and not scientific at all. But the subconscious can work in mysterious ways ...

The Stoic solution to all of this is to catch your strong emotions before they develop. This is a preventative approach. Rather than trying to manage out-of-control emotions, the goal is to deal with them before they get to that stage. We often have to act quickly though – sometimes we only have a few seconds before emotions take us over.

The Stoic philosopher Athenodorus Cananites spent time teaching philosophy to the Roman Emperor Octavian. One of his hot tips for dealing with anger was to recite the alphabet backwards before responding. This is the perfect example of inserting a wedge between what happens and how one reacts. Presumably, when someone would annoy Octavian, he would start recalling the alphabet backwards. I love this image!

It's actually very useful advice. Taking a break gives us time to calm down from the initial shock. Remember, those *propatheiai* emotions can be tempting to engage with. However, our goal is to avoid stoking the fire. Delaying our response can massively impact how we handle our emotions. Slowly counting to 10, singing the National Anthem, reciting your favourite Stoic quotes or recalling the backwards alphabet will all work well. The simple act of hesitating before giving a response can make a huge difference.

There's nothing worse than hastily replying to an email in an angry state of mind. You can end up saying something that you regret and the whole situation can spiral out of control. Taking time so that you can reply with a measured response is the Stoic solution. A small break can change everything.

Another tactic that the Stoics advise us to use when facing strong emotions is to embrace philosophy. Seneca recommends that when struck with grief, seeking out philosophy can bring us comfort. A lot of the time, this philosophy refers to our ability to reason. The Stoics absolutely loved reason and saw it as an incredible tool for dealing with our *passions*. By working with reason, we can have a better understanding of what is actually going on.

If something bad happens to us, we can feel upset. But if we add an additional narrative of how we wish we could change something or if only we had done this or that, we can torment ourselves. Knowing that we can't control what happens to us allows us to relax – we really don't have to be so hard on ourselves. Life can be tough but we can choose how we respond to it. That's how we get our power back ... The Stoic Golden Rule comes to the rescue again!

Using logic and reasoning when dealing with strong emotions is exactly what a lot of modern therapies suggest that we do. REBT and CBT are based on this and both address issues ranging from social anxiety to depression. These therapies focus on the internal dialogue we use and we can see the influence that Stoicism has had here – using logic can help us to break the illusions and stories that we tell ourselves. We can be our own worst enemies when it comes to emotions, but logic and reasoning can help us to shatter these illusions. Viva La Logica! Or something like that.

ALTERNATIVE WAYS TO MANAGE EMOTIONS

There are two ideas that I like to use in my life when dealing with powerful emotions. Interestingly, they are contradictory – one encourages us to distract ourselves from what we are feeling and the other encourages us to investigate what we are feeling. These ideas have helped me when dealing with anxiety, nerves, sadness and anger. And a whole host of other emotions. They are powerful and effective. See what you think.

DISTRACTION

When we start to feel overwhelmed with emotion, distracting ourselves can work wonders. If we engage the logical part of our brains, this can be an effective way for us to manage powerful waves of emotion. Games like chess, Tetris and sudoku all require the logical part of the brain to kick into gear. It's pretty hard for both the logical and emotional parts of the brain to be firing at the same time, so if we start stimulating our minds with puzzles and games that demand logic, we notice a significant shift in our mindsets. In a way, you can think of this as a combination of the Stoic suggestion of delaying emotional responses and employing logic/reasoning at the same time. Two for the price of one – bonus! (As a side note – Tetris can be a great way to deal with a panic attack. I've used this before and it has helped me to settle my panic.)

Another alternative here is to do something physical. If possible, when you feel strong emotions building up, start doing something that engages your body: press-ups, sprints, squats, etc. You have loads of options. It's probably worth mentioning that this will greatly depend upon the situation. If your boss comes over to you and says something that really winds you up, instantly sprinting off into the distance might not go down too well. Common sense with all of this is advised.

Distracting yourself as a form of managing emotions works well but it won't necessarily address the root cause of problems. Sometimes there might not be a root cause and you'll just want to manage a difficult moment in time. In other instances, there might be a specific trigger for your problem, so it's not a bad idea to investigate what's going on.

INVESTIGATION

Paying attention to what we're experiencing can be empowering. There's a therapy called ACT, which, although not

Stoic in origin, has some important ideas that support the Stoic concept of learning how to manage emotion.

ACT stands for Acceptance and Commitment Therapy and is all about mindfully being aware of what strong emotions actually feel like within our bodies. By paying attention to the specific sensations associated with different emotions, and accepting them, we can learn to let them just be there. When we try to mask these emotions, it can feel unpleasant.

Fully embracing any discomfort associated with these emotions can change our relationship with them. If you stare at these feelings and observe them closely, they often lose their power. A practical example will help to illustrate this better …

If you have an ice bath, it's an incredibly painful experience. However, if you mindfully focus on the pain, it changes. It actually becomes more bearable if you acknowledge the sensations and let your body feel them. For example, try exploring the sharpness of the cold in your mind inquisitively. This is counter-intuitive but it works. I know, it sounds crazy! I wouldn't have believed it until I tried it. By investigating the physical sensations, we experience them in a different way.

This is the same for emotions. If we feel them fully, we can learn to accept them. Anger might feel hot in your chest. Fear might feel like bubbling in your stomach. Frustration might feel like tightness in your jaw. There are many ways that these emotions present themselves and they will likely be different for each of us. When we accept them, our brains will eventually get bored with these sensations and can relax a little. Suddenly we find it easier to let strong emotions go.

This is obviously much easier to write about than to put into practice but there is a specific technique that's particularly helpful with all of this. It's called RAIN:

R – Recognize
Recognize the emotion/sensation you are feeling.

A – Accept
Accept that you are feeling this way.

I – Investigate
Spend time exploring the sensation. Let your mind focus on all of the different physical components of it.

N – Non-attachment
Let it go! Don't attach labels to the whole situation. It is what it is. And it will pass.

Here's an example dialogue of me dealing with pre-climb nerves on a route that looks scary. These are the kind of nerves where it feels very intense and you can feel adrenaline in your body. Shaky knee kind of stuff.

Step 1 – Recognize
"Right, this climb looks scary. Hmm. Feeling ... a ... bit ... nervous ..."

Step 2 – Accept
"OK, this is normal. These feelings are part of the process."

Step 3 – Investigate
"What does it feel like? Well ... My mouth feels dry. My palms are sweaty. My heart rate is up. I feel a little nauseous. I feel small and quiet."

Step 4 – Non-attachment
"Let this go. These feelings will pass – you are not these feelings. They are temporary. Time to climb."

At this point I'll proceed to climb the route effortlessly with tons of style or the climb won't go to plan. Either way, the process of dealing with the pre-nerves and embracing powerful emotions can help this moment in time be less intense.

Another way to take investigation further is to explore the actual reasons behind why you might be experiencing these powerful emotions in the first place. If it's things like feeling apprehensive about a work presentation, that's pretty obvious. But if you're experiencing serious and constant rage over tiny things or experiencing a lot of sadness within your life, exploring the reasons for this can help you to manage them. A professional therapist might be advisable at this point. There are plenty of psychology books that you could look into here too. Exploring this goes beyond the realms of this book (as there are many potential reasons for these powerful emotions being triggered) but it's worth pointing out that you have options.

THE STOIC GUIDE TO EMOTIONS

I'd like to share with you a brief guide to dealing with some common emotions – the Stoic way. I've created a list of negative emotions and given you some ideas from Stoicism that can help you to manage them. I'd suggest testing them out and seeing what helps you when your *passions* become overwhelming.

ANGER

According to Seneca: *"The greatest remedy for anger is delay."* So, the next time you feel that rage creeping in … STOP! Give yourself some time before you react. Don't add fuel to the fire. Make sure that you disconnect from the intensity of the moment and focus on how you respond to the situation. Maybe, like Octavian, you can test out the backwards alphabet trick.

FEAR/ANXIETY

Aurelius suggests that our perceptions play a huge role in anxiety and fear – *"Today I escaped anxiety. Or no, I discarded it, because it was within me, in my own perceptions – not outside."* So, the next time you start feeling afraid or anxious, lean into logic. Use reasoning to question this fear and check your perceptions. Is your anxiety based on reality? Or your imagination?

GRIEF

Seneca puts it succinctly when he says: *"The grief that has been conquered by reason is calmed forever."* So when facing a sad situation, rely on reasoning. The Stoic Golden Rule and focusing on what you can and can't control will be particularly helpful here. Pay attention to what you can do right now and willingly accept the things over which you have no power.

JEALOUSY

Aurelius has some brilliant advice for us when we're starting to feel a little jealous, greedy and ungrateful for what we have in life: *"Don't set your mind on things you don't possess ... but count the blessings you actually possess and think how much you would desire them if they weren't already yours."* Gratitude for what you have is the answer to jealousy for the things you don't have.

FINAL THOUGHTS

Being a Stoic doesn't mean that you aren't emotional. Not at all. Being a Stoic suggests that you are able to manage powerful emotions effectively when they crop up. And let's face it, that's going to be a lot. After all, life can be very unpredictable. I think it's really important to remember this distinction because so many people mess this bit up when they talk about Stoicism. It's a common mistake to label Stoics as emotionless. I'm tempted to start a range of bumper stickers saying: "Stoics have feelings too".

We should embrace our emotions but not let them be in control of us. I think Aurelius' words will conclude this principle nicely:

"How satisfying it is to dismiss and block out any upsetting or foreign impression, and immediately to have peace in all things."
Marcus Aurelius

PRACTICAL EXERCISES

The purpose of these exercises is to help control overwhelming emotions.

COUNT TO 10 (AND THEN AGAIN)
When dealing with strong and overwhelming emotions and a desire to react, delay everything. Count to 10. Then do it again. Recite the alphabet backwards or a specific phrase that you've come up with (anything long will work here). The goal is to delay things for as long as possible.

Call to action – when someone angers you or you feel strong emotions building up, create a wedge of time and don't engage with anything for a short while. Make notes in your journal and try to collect three examples of this happening. Write about what happened, how it felt and what was the outcome.

RAIN

A great way to deal with strong emotions is to use the RAIN exercise from ACT:

Recognize/Accept/Investigate/Non-attachment

In essence, if you focus on the physical sensations associated with your strong emotions, you can interact with them in a different way and learn to become a conscious observer of your feelings – rather than getting completely caught up in them. A full explanation of the technique can be found earlier in the principle (page 119). Test it out and see how you get on.

LOGIC YOUR WAY OUT OF TROUBLE

This exercise is built on the CBT technique of questioning all of your negative thoughts. When strong emotions pop up, use logic and reasoning to question them. The Stoics believed that philosophy was the cure for everything and this type of logical enquiring was popular. Have a go at leaning into logic when you feel emotional. Question everything you think. Now journal about your experiences.

DISTRACTION TACTICS

When feeling overwhelmed, a distraction tactic avoids letting those emotions overwhelm us. Games like Tetris/logic-based games/crosswords/chess/sudoku, etc. can be a fantastic way to get you out of the emotional part of your mind and into the logical part of your mind. So download some apps on your phone and test them out when things start getting intense.

THE EMOTIONAL DETECTIVE

This exercise requires you to look deeper into the root causes of your strong emotions. This is essentially an investigation into the underlying emotional issues. Looking at your whole life and asking yourself if you are balanced in all areas can be difficult, but the growth that can come from addressing imbalances can be profound. The use of a therapist or reading specific books on tough emotions is a good place to start.

JOURNALING PROMPTS

Your journaling exercise for this principle is to reflectively write about the emotions you encounter throughout the day. Is there a particular one that keeps cropping up? Is there something that you always find difficult to deal with? The goal with all of this is to spend some time thinking about what emotions you tend to lean toward. We all experience different emotions depending upon our circumstances, but on a day-to-day basis, we often have dominant emotions. When you've figured out what this is, test out some of the Stoic coping strategies I've mentioned earlier. Work through my suggested exercises and see which help when facing powerful emotions. Take notes about what happened.

10

PRINCIPLE 8: DEALING WITH OTHERS

"The tranquillity that comes when you stop caring what they say. Or think, or do. Only what you do."

Marcus Aurelius

SUMMARY OF PRINCIPLE

The world is a diverse place and we must be prepared to encounter different points of view. People will say things that we don't like, but we can deal with this in a philosophically mature way.

PRINCIPLE

We live in a world with incredible diversity. We have a huge mix of cultures, environments and ideas all floating around on this planet. It's one of the most beautiful things about existence in my opinion. Variety is the spice of life and all that. The unfortunate thing is, these differences often end up clashing. Opposing ideas can cause massive problems. And I don't just mean the classic Marmite debate here ... We only need to briefly look at human history to see what a difference of opinion can lead to – war, famine, torture, death, destruction, hatred and anger.

The modern world is packed with people who think differently than we do. Polarization is real and there are great divides in the way people see the world, and we don't have to look far to find examples of this. In reality, it's not so much the divide that's the problem, it's how we handle that divide. Stoicism has a lot to say about all of this.

The Stoics aspired to cultivate a philanthropic attitude toward humankind and an inclusive approach to dealing with others. A "we're all in this together" sort of attitude. The idea can be summed up by the Aurelius quote:

"What's bad for the hive is bad for the bee."

Marcus Aurelius

That is, if we aren't good to each other, it's going to come back around and bite us from behind. Caring for humanity and our fellow citizens is seen as an important part of Stoic ethics. It's something that enables us to be better individuals and helps us to build a better world.

Zeno, the founder of Stoicism, wrote a book called *The Republic* (often referred to as *Zeno's Republic*). Unfortunately, this has been lost in the depths of time and no copies exist today. What we do know about the book is that his ideal republic was seen as an enlightened group of friends – a world of equality and friendship.

Inclusivity is an integral part of Stoic ethics. It stems from a technical concept called *oikeiôsis* – a word that's quite tricky to translate. I'll do my best ... The idea of *oikeiôsis* is that we perceive something as our own. The word "affinity" or "belonging" could be used here. The Stoic Hierocles did a pretty good job of explaining it with his famous concentric circles example. So, let's start with this …

The idea is fairly simple. Our relationship with everyone can be seen as concentric circles. There are several circles. At the centre we have ourselves. In the next circle we have our family. The next one has our friends and extended family in it. The next one is our fellow citizens – people who live in the same town as us. We then have a circle filled with people who live in the same country as us. And finally, we have a circle that encompasses all of humanity. Here's a diagram:

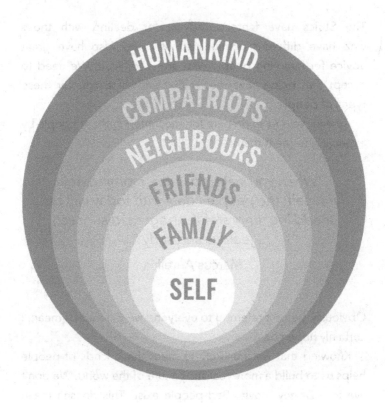

The goal of *oikeiôsis* is to bring all of these circles closer to the centre; to bring everyone closer to us so that we care for humanity with more depth and empathy. (Yes, this also includes your really weird neighbour; this is about bringing people together.)

Basically, if we view others as fellow citizens of the universe, we're starting in the right place. Even if we have a difference of opinion, there is common ground. We are all humans. Having said all of this, we are still likely to meet difficult people in our lives. Thankfully, the Stoics have some pragmatic tips for dealing with them.

HOW TO DEAL WITH DIFFICULT PEOPLE

The Stoics have fantastic advice for dealing with those who have different opinions to us. They also have great advice for handling people who are ... difficult. We need to accept that being alive means that we will encounter these types of people.

Aurelius tells us to prepare for encountering these people by expecting to meet them:

"When you wake up in the morning, tell yourself: the people I deal with today will be meddling, ungrateful, arrogant, dishonest, jealous and surly."

Marcus Aurelius

Obviously, he isn't referring to everyone we will meet. I mean, I certainly hope not.

Knowing that we are likely to meet these kinds of people helps us to build a more realistic picture of the world. We don't live in a Disney movie. Bad people exist. This doesn't mean that we have to think everyone is awful and that the world is a horrible and cruel place where everyone conspires against us (this would also be an unrealistic view of reality) – it's about building an awareness that there are difficult people out there. We can still have an inclusive attitude and see them as fellow citizens of the universe – but we don't have to endorse their behaviour or mindsets.

Aurelius goes on to say how their poor judgement causes them to behave in this way. And although they see the world from a different perspective, they are still similar to us in nature and therefore we need to remember that they can change. There is still good in them.

"They are like this because they can't tell good from evil. But I have seen the beauty of good, and the ugliness of evil and have recognized that the wrongdoer has a nature related to my own – not of the same blood or birth, but the same mind, and possessing a share of the divine."

Marcus Aurelius

Looking for what we have in common with people rather than our differences is a great place to start. We might have to zoom out and focus on the fact that we are both human (this will be true for particularly challenging people) and take things from there. But, focusing on how we are similar can be a good footing for negotiations.

So, we've accepted that difficult people are out there. We've accepted that they are citizens of the universe and they are in essence like us – they are human ... But what do we actually do when we encounter one of these people? What do we do when their behaviour is unacceptable? How do we manage this? How do we not punch someone in the face who clearly deserves it? Well, luckily, we have options ...

The Stoics valued character highly. How we deal with difficult people says a lot about our character. Rather than worrying about what they are saying or doing, though, we need to focus on our response to their actions. This is the only thing we can control. The Stoic Golden Rule is back again.

We can't control what someone else thinks or does. We can try to influence their thoughts and behaviour but what they actually end up thinking or doing isn't up to us. If we care too much, we are not treating the situation as an *indifference* (which we should). What people think about us and how they behave around us is up to them. We can still be a decent human being irrespective of what they do.

If someone is awful to us, we can choose how we respond to this. If we can learn to forgive these people, we show true strength of character. Their poor behaviour is a reflection of their weak character and the Stoics would encourage us to feel sorry for them. They are not in control of their minds. They lack discipline. We do not need to sink to their level and we do not need to mirror their bad behaviour by acting poorly ourselves. We can be disciplined with our actions and turn a challenging encounter with someone into a test of our character.

"For to scheme how to bite back the biter and to return evil for evil is the act not of a human being but of a wild beast."
Musonius Rufus

EMPATHY

The Stoics encourage us to seek forgiveness and see the good in people. A great way to do this is to increase our empathy toward others. And the way we increase our empathy is to look at things from a different perspective.

My wife, Helen, is incredibly good at doing this. She is highly empathetic and is always thinking about other people. She's a very caring person and I admire this quality in her. Whenever someone is driving like a complete plonker, Helen always tries to look at things from a different perspective. She'll say things like, "Maybe they are racing to get to the hospital," or, "Maybe they are distracted by bad news." This type of response isn't natural to me – if someone is driving like a psychopath, I find it hard to think of them in this light. I'm normally straight on the horn … But that doesn't help the situation. To be fair, I'm getting better at relaxing and letting things go. I'm following Helen the Stoic's example.

The psychology behind this thinking is sound. As human beings we tend to undervalue the influence of a stressful situation on others. We don't know what has happened to them to cause them to behave like this. It's easy for us to judge someone's bad behaviour but most of the time we don't have access to the full context. We don't have to agree with what they are doing or even like it, but by thinking about things from this perspective, we can bring empathy into the equation.

A great way to consider this is to remember how quickly we can forgive our friends when they do something bad or something that we disapprove of. We will often excuse their behaviour, claiming they are under a lot of pressure or that x/y/z has probably caused them to do this. Interestingly, we tend to do the opposite with people we don't know. When someone does something awful, we assume that this is their character – that their disposition made them do it. In reality, we don't know what they are like as people and we don't know the full picture.

This type of thinking can help us to cultivate *oikeiôsis* and to develop an affinity for those around us, even when we don't like what they are doing. People are more than their weakest moment and we must remember this.

DEALING WITH CRITICS

The Stoics have fantastic advice for dealing with critics. And there are of plenty of those critics out there! You know the type … You tell them a good piece of news and they find a way to turn it into a negative. Whatever you do or say, they will criticize it or put a negative spin on it. "Oh – you're having a kid! Well, don't expect to sleep ever again. My life ended when I had kids. Former shell of myself now. But, congratulations!"

It doesn't matter what you talk to them about, there will always be some reason to complain. Moaning. Criticizing. It's exhausting just thinking about all of that negativity! We all know these people. There's one word for them. Toxic. It's best to avoid them or at least reduce the amount of time you spend with them.

A funny exercise that highlights how ludicrously critical these people can be is to go on TripAdvisor and look at the 1-star reviews of incredible locations around the world. The Eiffel Tower … the Leaning Tower of Pisa … Niagara Falls … ALL RUBBISH! Whatever the sight, you can almost guarantee that there's going to be a 1-star review written by a critic. The Matterhorn is too pointy. The Grand Canyon is too hot and doesn't have any toilets. The Mona Lisa is too small. The Northern Lights are rubbish and didn't come out at 8:53pm on January 23rd. The pyramids are too old and were a bit too sandy. Mount Fuji doesn't have a lift to the top.

I feel like a lot of these people are ready to talk to the manager … Alas, we must accept that there are these sorts of people in society and we have to learn to live with them. The best thing we can do is not weight their opinions in reality.

Of course, if what they are saying might be of use to us, then we can take the feedback on board and use it to improve our characters – Great! But if it's unhelpful and malicious criticism that's not coming from a place of constructive advice, we would be wise to ignore their words completely.

"It never ceases to amaze me: we love ourselves more than other people, but care more about their opinion than our own."

Marcus Aurelius

FINAL THOUGHTS

Throughout our lives we will have relationships with many different people. This will range from professional to personal and will encompass a huge range of personalities. One of the best things we can do is prepare to meet people we are going to find difficult and challenging. This is an inevitability. Awkward people are going to crop up in our lives and we must be able to manage them. The following six steps can be used as a way to Stoically handle these people:

1. Accept that you're going to meet difficult people.
2. Feel sorry for their weakness of character.
3. See your encounter as a test of your character.
4. Picture them in a kind light – use the loving kindness meditation in the practical exercises section to build empathy.
5. Think about your common humanity – not the individual who is being difficult.
6. Forgive them.

Taking these Stoic steps will allow you to deal with the most challenging of people. I wish you the best of luck! Oh, and while you're at it, keep Aurelius' words in mind:

"Does someone despise me? That's their problem. Mine is to ensure that what I do or say does not deserve sneer. Does someone hate me? Again, it is their problem. My job is to be friendly and charitable to everyone including those who hate me and show them their mistake."

Marcus Aurelius

PRACTICAL EXERCISES

The purpose of these exercises is to help us deal with difficult people and to make us feel more connected with humanity.

IT'S NOT ME, IT'S YOU
This exercise is about staying in control when someone is rude, unkind or unpleasant to you. Slow down and delay extreme responses while you give yourself time to think. View it as a test of YOUR character – a mini challenge – and treat every time you get insulted as an opportunity to grow and practise your response. Journal about your experiences.

CITIZEN OF THE UNIVERSE
For this exercise I'd like to encourage you to partake in random acts of kindness. Examples include buying a stranger a coffee/ letting someone go in front of you in a queue/holding the door open for someone/donating time and money to charity/giving

random compliments to people. Be creative and come up with your own random acts of kindness.

By focusing on being an active member of the community and distributing kindness, you are helping to make the world a better place. It's a small step but starting with our own behaviour is a great beginning.

The Stoics saw themselves as citizens of the universe – equality and kindness for all, even toward the difficult people. Try to apply this concept to your life and see yourself as a part of humanity and a citizen of the universe too.

EMPATHY

A great exercise for exploring this can be found in Buddhism. It's called Loving Kindness Meditation. Yes, I know this isn't Stoic but it's an amazing way to increase empathy and complements our Stoic practice nicely. By wishing someone that has wronged you well, you can let go of the animosity you feel toward them. Here's the exercise:

Firstly, picture someone you deeply care about. Now wish them well. Wish them happiness and picture them filled with joy. Spend a few minutes doing this. Really build a clear picture in your head of what this looks like. Imagine them in different scenarios being happy. Picture them as a child playing. Picture them on their wedding day (even if they aren't married – don't worry about the details). Picture them surrounded by their family. Be creative and whiz through moments in their life and imagine them being happy.

Next, do the exact same exercise but for someone you don't know well. Spend some time wishing them well and send positive vibes in their direction. After you've done this, think of someone you find difficult. Someone that you have strong negative feelings toward. Now wish them well. Run through the exercise and picture them being happy. This can be hard. Stick with the exercise and see what happens. Did the way you think about that person change at all? Did you see them in a different light? This practice can be used to build empathy and can be highly effective. I find it particularly difficult doing the exercise with certain people but that shows me that there's a lot for me to get out of it. I still have room to grow and there's space for me to increase my compassion.

MORE THAN THEIR WEAKEST MOMENT

This exercise can be used to soften your dislike for someone. When someone behaves badly, try to think of the reasons that might be driving their behaviour. Maybe something has happened in their personal life – they might have recently lost a relative or partner. Try to picture as many alternative reasons for this person acting badly as possible.

The goal of this exercise is to put all of this in context and appreciate that everyone has moments of weakness. Remember, they are more than just this moment.

You don't have to spend extra time with this person but you don't want to hold onto hatred for them – this just makes you unhappy or unbalanced. By running through this visualization exercise, you can soften your dislike for someone and learn to let go. The results can be liberating.

DEBATE TIME

Deliberately seek out someone with a different opinion on something and try to remain as calm as possible while you debate with them. Talking calmly to someone who disagrees with you is a great measure of how in control of your emotions you are.

Whether a debating club or Twitter, or just chatting to your opinionated friend about something you both disagree on – there are many options for putting yourself in hostile environments. Give it a go and see how you get on.

JOURNALING PROMPTS

Your journaling exercise for this principle is to reflect on the difficult people in your life. Write a list of people that you struggle with and start testing out these Stoic exercises on them. What happened? Did it help looking for the common humanity in both of you? Did you try out the Loving Kindness Meditation? How hard was that exercise?

Make a note each time you encounter difficult and unreasonable behaviour and grade your response. If you managed to keep your cool and actually turned the situation around, give yourself an A. Try to get better grades as you respond to difficult people out in the real world. Pay attention to what helped you and what didn't. Add all of this to your journal and look for themes.

11

PRINCIPLE 9:
MEMENTO MORI

"Let us prepare our minds as if we'd come to the very end of life. Let us postpone nothing. Let us balance life's books each day. The one who puts the finishing touches on their life each day is never short of time."

Seneca

WARNING

This is an advanced Stoic concept. It can be extremely difficult for some people to use and, if done incorrectly, it can put you in a negative mental space. Be particularly careful with this if you are experiencing anxiety, depression or any other mental health conditions. Feel free to skip the principle if it's too much. You can always come back to it at a later stage.

SUMMARY OF PRINCIPLE

Contemplating our own mortality helps us to increase our gratitude for life. It can also help us to live with more presence of mind and a clearer sense of purpose and direction.

PRINCIPLE

The Stoics spent a lot of time writing and talking about death. It's an important theme in the philosophy and something they regularly thought about. This wasn't meant to be a gloomy and morbid exercise but a way of increasing their gratitude for life. It was also a great way to keep their egos in check.

Aurelius, the Roman Emperor and arguably the most powerful human on the planet at the time, would often reflect on his own mortality. He constantly referenced this in *Meditations* and used the exercise as a way to stay humble. With all of that power, it would have been easy for him to feel invincible. Reminding himself that he would die helped him to keep in touch with reality.

The Latin phrase *memento mori* means – "remember you are mortal". It's something that the Stoics would regularly use. In fact, it wasn't just the Stoics; Roman generals would have *memento mori* whispered into their ears when appointed to a new position of power. It was a way to keep them grounded. In all honesty, I don't think it would go down too well if Helen came home and started talking about a promotion at work and I went up to her and whispered, "That's great darling, but don't forget you're still going to die."

It might sound blunt or crass to talk about death in the modern world but should this really be the case? It's intriguing that death is such a taboo topic, particularly in the West. The reality is, it's something that we all have to face, whether we like it or not. Having said that, there are some people who are desperately trying to beat death by freezing their brains or trying to create technology that will keep them alive. But, for now, immortality is something that sits comfortably in the science-fiction section of the bookstore. This means that we all need to accept that we are one day going to die.

For some, the denial of death is a serious problem. The horrors of non-existence can cause people a lot of mental distress. I've personally found it difficult to think about dying in the past. Avoiding thinking about it doesn't solve the problem though. Eventually, we have to face the facts. If we leave it for too long, it can grow into something overwhelming – anyone up for an existential crisis? Sometimes we have to sit down and stare reality in the eyes. Or death, as it might be in this case.

DEATH MEDITATION

The Stoics thought that it was our fear of death that was worse than death itself. Epictetus highlights this:

> *"... It's the fear of pain and death we need to fear."*

Epictetus

This sentiment is also mirrored by other Stoics. The idea is that death isn't bad – because it's a natural event. However, an irrational fear toward it is bad. We need to learn to make peace with death and accept that it's something we are all going to have to deal with. This is no easy task, but the Stoics have a very specific way to do this – meditating on death.

A death meditation is essentially time spent contemplating our own mortality. This can be a powerful exercise and something that can genuinely help us to bring a deeper sense of gratitude into our lives.

How does it bring us gratitude and a deeper sense of purpose? Well, thinking about not being alive instantly makes us feel grateful for actually being alive. Life is very precious but we often forget this. We get stuck into a daily routine and think that everything is always going to stay the same. This is an illusion that the death meditation helps us to overcome.

Think about the countless number of people who have a brush with death and suddenly change the course of their life. It happens all the time. For example, someone in a bad car accident realizes that they don't love their job and that their life is not what they wanted it to be. This realization can cause them to change direction. They become acutely aware that time is finite. Suddenly, there is a desire to live with more purpose and direction. The death meditation can be used to kick that motivation into gear without a specific event or close call as the trigger. Handy, right?

Contemplating death is very much the next step to negative visualization (Principle 6). Not only can it help us to be grateful, but also to psychologically prepare. There are many ways that we can participate in a death meditation, so I'll suggest a few options to explore.

It's worth putting in a little note of caution here too. Spending time thinking about your mortality is hard and challenging work. It might also bring up some serious issues that will require working through with a therapist. If you find that you begin to obsess over death and have suicidal thoughts while using these exercises, speak to someone immediately. Pay attention to your mind and don't let this concept spiral out of control.

Here are a variety of ways you can contemplate your own death:

1. Picture your funeral.
   Imagine that you are a fly on the wall at your funeral.
   Picture yourself lying in a coffin surrounded by friends and
   family. What sort of things would people say? What stories
   would they tell? Who would be there? Explore the details

of the event in your mind and then make notes on how it made you feel.

2. Think about what happens after you die.
Spend some time thinking about where you go after you die. This will likely be different depending upon who you are. For example, if you have a religion in your life, you will have a different take than an atheist. Explore as many different possibilities as you can imagine. This can be a tough thing to think about and can make your mind spin. I'll talk about what the Stoics thought about this later.

3. Think about what happened before you were born.
Have a go at contemplating where you were before you were born. Is this the same place that you will return to when you die? What did this non-existence feel like? Is pre-birth easier or harder to comprehend than death?

4. Imagine a world without you in it.
Spend some time thinking about somewhere that you don't live. Maybe imagine Paris (if you live in Paris, choose a different city). Now think about how that city is existing just fine without you there. People are out on the streets going about their business. Restaurants have customers. Schools have children. Where are you in this picture? Exactly! You aren't there. Life goes on. Now imagine a world where you aren't in it. Does this make you more grateful for the experience you are having right now? Or does it scare you?

5. Picture the actual process of dying.
What do you think that would feel like? This doesn't have to be graphic, although it can be. Visually imagine taking your last breath. What do you think will happen? What will this feel like? Imagine a variety of different ways that you might die ... OK, this is pretty intense so take it easy with this.

Use a timer to work on these thought experiments and focus on exploring each idea as much as possible in the time limit. Maybe try five minutes for each and work through them systematically.

This isn't going to be easy but it can be a profound experience if you get it right. If you get it wrong and start feeling terrible, you can always revisit my "HELP – What to do if you get sucked into a black hole of despair" section in the Negative Visualization principle. This works in the same way for a death meditation and can help you to ground yourself in the present. Plus, a comedic distraction is a great way to help you snap out of spiralling thoughts. Memes anyone?

The Stoics would use this contemplative practice daily. The morning or evening would be used as a time to do a little death meditating. Seneca recommends that we wake up and treat the day as if it was our last. Imagine how that would affect our thinking and behaviour. He then goes on to recommend that we tell ourselves that "we may not wake up" each evening before we go to sleep. Constant awareness of our mortality helps us to act with purpose. Rufus succinctly states:

> "It is not possible to live well today unless you treat it as your last day."
>
> Musonius Rufus

I've personally used this idea a lot and now regularly think about my own death. When I was particularly anxious I wouldn't have been able to go anywhere near this exercise. No way! But now that I have changed my relationship with anxiety and understand myself a lot better, it's something that I use all the time. I have first-hand experience of how powerful it can be and know that it's an extremely practical way to reflect on how I'm living my life.

THE LAST TIME

We have no idea when we are going to die. It could be today, tomorrow or many years from now in the distant future. The truth is, we just don't know. Because we don't know, the Stoics advise us to act as if we might leave this life at any minute. Aurelius puts it like this:

> *"You could leave life right now. Let that determine what you do and say and think."*
>
> Marcus Aurelius

If you think that you might die later today, would you still want to have that argument with your spouse? Would you still want to be rude to a colleague? This would be the last time they saw you – the last time you were alive would have been spent being awful to someone else. Would you want that to be your legacy? Would you still want to blow five hours on Netflix? Or would you get out into the real world to appreciate your last sunset?

By becoming conscious of the fact that we might die at any minute, we have a heightened appreciation for what we are doing in the moment. Right here, right now. This can be a useful way to live a more present existence.

I like the idea of creating a list of mundane things that range from taking out the bins to washing up and applying this idea to them. This might be the last time I ever do the activity, so it helps me to frame it differently. It also really helps to enhance the good stuff. When you experience something lovely, reflect that this might be the last time you ever experience it. This can help us to really savour the moment.

ON PURPOSE

The other bonus gained from reflecting on the fact that we could die at any minute is that it naturally encourages us to think about how we are spending our time. If this was my last day on Earth, would I really want to spend it doing this?

Thinking about how we use our time can be very powerful. Considering that we spend a third of our life asleep, a huge chunk of it at work and a bunch of it doing trivial tasks, we can often be left wondering what time we actually have left. Are we spending it wisely?

Living with purpose and meaning is something that can help us to feel satisfied with life. Consider the following juicy questions ... What am I doing with my life? Am I pleased with the direction I am heading? What are my values? Am I living a good life?

Do any of these have a sense of urgency to them? Well, if you are acutely aware that you might die tomorrow, these important questions suddenly become a real priority. That's the power of *memento mori*. There's nothing quite like a reminder that you are going to die. It's a great way to get motivated!

A life well-lived is one where we spend time doing things that have meaning and value. The Stoics argue that it doesn't matter how long we live, but that we use our time wisely. Enter Seneca:

"It's not at all that we have too short a time to live, but that we squander a great deal of it. Life is long enough, and it's given in sufficient measure to do many great things if we spend it well. But when poured down the drain of luxury and neglect, when it's employed to no good end, we're finally driven to see that it has passed by before we even recognize it

*passing. And so it is – we don't receive a short
life, we make it so."*

Seneca

Invest some energy in thinking about your time. Are you spending it well? Maybe you should dust off that old bucket list or write a new one. We don't know how long we have, so we need to seize the day.

THE STOICS' THOUGHTS ON DEATH

*"Death, like birth, is just a natural process,
material elements combining, growing, decaying
and finally separating and completely dispersing."*

Marcus Aurelius

So, what did the Stoics actually think about death. Well, they saw death as part of nature and therefore didn't view it as a negative thing. You've seen *The Lion King*, surely?! The circle of life and all that ... Well, the Stoics saw it like that. Nature is doing its thing. Death is a natural part of life. Without death, we have no life. It's nothing to be feared.

The Stoics believed that whatever happens to us after we die is something that we have no control over so we shouldn't let it worry us. They were typically agnostic to the idea of an afterlife and the immortality of the soul. However, they tended to think that we would return back to nature when we die and go to the place we were before we were born. That's pretty difficult to contemplate, right? Spending time thinking about where you were before you were born can be challenging. It's something that our minds struggle to comprehend (well, mine does anyway). That's why I think it's an interesting exercise to explore in the death meditation mentioned earlier. Contemplating this can help us to get closer to how the Stoics viewed death – the same as pre-birth.

A VISUAL REMINDER OF
MEMENTO MORI

In Mexico, the Day of the Dead is a holiday where families and friends gather to celebrate those who have died. You've probably seen the elaborate skeleton costumes and funky face paint that people wear during the festivities. Mixed with bright colours, the festival looks so vibrant.

The icon of the Day of the Dead is *La Calavera Catrina*, the elegant female skeleton wearing a fancy hat. You will see beautiful variations of her throughout the celebrations as people dress in her style. The modern depiction of *La Catrina* was created by the artist José Guadalupe Posada. He was a political cartoonist that drew skeletons (*calaveras*) as a way to remind people of their mortality. *La Catrina* was created to represent the Mexicans that aspired to be wealthy and aristocratic. He wanted them to remember that no matter who you were, where you were from or how much money you had, you would still end up a skeleton. His famous quote, "Death is democratic" sums this up beautifully!

Skeletons and skulls are a visual reminder of where we are all heading. When we look at the bust of a skull, we are reminded that we will all eventually end up as a pile of bones. Having a reminder of this is not a bad thing. It can prompt us to live each moment in our lives as best we can. Some people have opted for a *memento mori* tattoo to help them remember this. Others have artwork in their homes as a reminder. I have a little Day of the Dead skull on my desk. It's colourful and reminds me of this concept whenever I look at it. I've given him a name. Cato.

Having a visual reminder of our mortality is the perfect way to keep this idea in our minds. Why not create your own reminder and see if it helps you to reflect on this Stoic principle?

FINAL THOUGHTS

We contemplate death to help us remove our fear of death. We also contemplate death to have a philosophical attitude toward it. This contemplation isn't done as a morbid exercise but to help us live with clarity, passion and purpose. Being aware of our mortality can be powerful and stop us from daydreaming our way through life.

It's very fitting that Aurelius' book *Meditations* ends with a note on death. He talks about accepting our fate and not begrudging the situation. We are encouraged to leave this life gracefully with philosophy in our minds. This seems like the perfect place to conclude the *memento mori* principle.

The last words in *Meditations*:

"You've lived as a citizen in a great city. Five years or a hundred – what's the difference? The Laws make no distinction. And to be sent away from it, not by a tyrant or a dishonest judge, but by Nature, who first invited you in – why is that so terrible? Like the impresario ringing down the curtain on an actor: 'But I've only gotten through three acts ...!' Yes. This will be a drama in three acts, the length fixed by the power that directed your creation, and now

*directs your dissolution. Neither was yours to
determine. So make your exit with grace – the
same grace shown to you."*
Marcus Aurelius

PRACTICAL EXERCISES

The purpose of the following exercises can be used to help us
appreciate our lives more.

DEATH MEDITATION
Spend some time contemplating your own mortality. As
mentioned earlier, use a timer and dedicate some attention to
the following thought experiments:

1. Picture your funeral.
2. Think about what happens after you die.
3. Think about what happened before you were born.
4. Imagine a world without you in it.
5. Picture the actual process of dying. What do you think that
   would feel like?

You can always revisit the death meditation section for
more specific prompts with all of this. I suggest taking notes
along the way.

CREATE A MORTALITY REMINDER
Create a visual representation of *memento mori* and carry it
around with you for a week. Maybe paint a Day of the Dead skull
or draw a little skeleton and put it on your desk. You have loads
of options for this and you can be creative with your designs.
If you're not feeling particularly arty or crafty, simply write the

words *memento mori* on a piece of paper and carry it around with you. Display it where you can see it and contemplate the message often.

THE BUCKET LIST

If today was your last day or year on Earth, what would you regret not doing? Spend some time creating a traditional bucket list and then think about how you can start attacking it. Death can be a real motivator!

THE LAST TIME LIST

We don't know when we are going to die so in theory everything we do could be the last time that we do it. The next time you do the following activities, consider that it might be the last time you do them:

1. Taking a shower
2. Opening your front door
3. Travelling to work

Be conscious of your actions and try to be present throughout the experience. The reason for this exercise is to help you live with more awareness of what you are doing.

To take all of this further, create your own Last Time List and use the actions as a trigger to be more present.

WHAT IS THE MEANING OF LIFE?

What is the meaning of your life? What are you here to do? What are your values? Are these the values you want to live your life by?

This exercise is all about finding a deeper meaning and purpose to life. Think deeply about the meaning of your life and explore this by writing down your ideas and talking about them to family and friends.

You could also start a meaning of life collection and begin interrogating everyone you know – ask them what they think the meaning of life is and make a note of their answers.

JOURNALING PROMPTS

Journaling on death can be tricky. I'd suggest using the thoughts and questions that come up during the death meditation as a good place to start. Record your concerns and then list the things that went well. There will likely be a lot of stuff going on in your mind when contemplating your own mortality so scribbling down your ideas can be cathartic.

I also think that focusing on the meaning of life can be a great way into journaling. Write down your values, start listing important questions that you want to explore and fill the page with notes. You can even collect what others say and add this to your journal.

12

PRINCIPLE 10:
THE COSMIC PERSPECTIVE

"You can discard most of the junk that clutters your mind ... and clear out space for yourself ... by comprehending the scale of the world ... by contemplating infinite time ... by thinking of the speed with which things change – each part of every thing; the narrow space between our birth and death; the infinite time before; the equally unbounded time that follows."

Marcus Aurelius

SUMMARY OF PRINCIPLE

By contemplating the vastness of the universe, we can bring perspective, gratitude and objectivity into our lives.

PRINCIPLE

Life is incredible. The chance of you being alive right now is so ridiculously small. If you stop to think about this fact, it can be truly mind-boggling. A number that gets thrown around a lot for this is 400 trillion to 1. That's insane! Even if this is an underestimation of the probability of being alive, it's still crazy.

Thinking about the odds is just the start though. By zooming out and looking at the bigger picture, we develop a different point of view. The Stoics encourage us to reflect on the grand scale of the universe, time, the scale of the world and the impermanent nature of existence as a way to bring objectivity and perspective to our lives. Thinking about these big ideas is beneficial as it can help us to feel more connected to the world around us. It helps us to feel part of something bigger. It's all too easy to get caught up in the minutia of day-to-day activities and a lot of this stuff is insignificant in the scheme of things. By becoming more aware of the miracle of our existence, we can learn to detach from unnecessary worries. Obviously, this is easier said than done, but thinking about the bigger picture can be a powerful practice.

SYMPATHEIA

There's an important concept in Stoicism called *sympatheia*. This is the idea that everything in the universe is interconnected. We are part of nature and not separate from it; we are made out of the same stuff as everything in existence. The scientist Carl Sagan describes it perfectly:

> *"The nitrogen in our DNA, the calcium in our teeth, the iron in our blood, the carbon in our apple pies were made in the interiors of collapsing stars. We are made of star stuff."*
> Carl Sagan

Our atoms have assumed many different forms since the dawn of time. In fact, the atoms inside your body right now might have been in a T-rex's toenail in the past. Jokes aside, the fact that we are all made of the same stuff can motivate us to strive for equality. When we break it down, we are all the same. All of us! It doesn't matter which country we are from, because, ultimately, we are citizens of the universe. We all come from the same place – stars! This is a beautiful concept.

Sympatheia encourages us to develop an inclusive world view. It's something that the Stoics highly valued and is as relevant today as it was 2,000 years ago. Contemplating our interconnectedness helps us to be better people. It makes us think about what we have in common rather than how we differ. In a world of polarization and division, this is something that we can all benefit from. It's an idea that brings us together and an idea that helps us to be kinder to each other.

THE VIEW FROM ABOVE

So, how can we put this into practice? Well, there's a classic Stoic exercise for this called "The View from Above". All we do is zoom out (in our minds) and look down at ourselves from above. And then we keep going!

You can give it a try now if you want ...

Imagine you are floating above your body and looking down. What does this look like? You can probably see the top of your head and everything that's around you. A cup of green tea? Nice! Now zoom out so that you're further up. What can you see? Roofs? Parks? Tiny ant-like people? Now go further. Maybe a few hundred metres more ... What can you see now? An entire town or city? Countryside? Zoom out further. What do you see? Your country? The curvature of the Earth? Go further! Now what? Planet Earth? Keep going ... What do you see? Our sun? Keep going! And now? The Milky Way? Keep going! Don't stop. What's there? AHHHHHHHH! The mind starts to melt as our tiny brains try to comprehend the vastness of the known universe.

Interestingly, a lot of astronauts report a feeling of greater connectedness with all of humanity after seeing Earth from space. Surrounded by emptiness and darkness, our planet looks lonely. We don't have any close neighbours and this lump of rock is all we have (for now, anyway). The Earth appears vulnerable and precious and needs us to take care of it. I can only imagine how powerful that experience would be. It must be incredibly profound to actually see the whole planet with your own eyes. Edgar Mitchell, the Apollo 14 astronaut and sixth person to walk on the moon, founded the Institute of Noetic Sciences (IONS) based on his experience of seeing the Earth from space and feeling a deep sense of connection to everything. His experience left a huge impression on him and when you read his explanation, it's the perfect description of the Stoic concept of *sympatheia*. After returning from space, Edgar spent the rest of his life exploring this experience from a scientific perspective. I recommend looking up his work.

I love learning about space and find it a truly fascinating subject. Whether it's reading about distant planets and galaxies or watching videos about how astronauts sleep in space (they float in sleeping bags tied to the wall, in case you were wondering), I can't get enough of it. The simple exercise of looking at some space stats and photos can be a wonderful way to experience this connection. It certainly helps me to get a strong sense of *sympatheia*. Give it a try.

IMPERMANENCE

Life equals constant change. Everything in the world around us is in a constant state of flux and movement. Nothing lasts forever. The idea of impermanence is an important theme in

Stoic philosophy and you'll notice it throughout the ancient texts. Aurelius references it loads and reflects on it frequently:

"Constantly reflect on how swiftly all that exists and is coming to be is swept past us and disappears from sight. For substance is like a river in perpetual flow, and its activities are ever changing, and its causes infinite in their variations, and hardly anything at all stands still; and ever at our side is the immeasurable span of the past and the yawning gulf of the future, into which all things vanish away. Then how is he not a fool who in the midst of all this is puffed up with pride, or tormented, or bewails his lot as though his troubles will endure for any great while?"

Marcus Aurelius

The Stoics were inspired by the ancient Greek philosopher Heraclitus. He was around before the Stoics (535–475 BCE) and was known for his work on impermanence. The two quotes that are attributed to him that concisely summarize his thoughts on change are:

"You could not step twice into the same river."
"Everything changes and nothing stands still."

Heraclitus

He also established the term "logos" which you will encounter if you read the Stoics. The term refers to the source and order of the cosmos. So, it's fair to say that he influenced the way that the Stoics thought about things. You can even see the direct influence on Aurelius with the river example in the quote earlier.

It's not hard to accept that change plays an important role in the world we live in today, but we easily forget this. We quickly despair over situations that will inevitably end at some point.

Dealing with mundane tasks is the perfect example of this ... We're not going to be doing them forever, but when we're in the middle of them, it's easy for us to get caught up in the situation. We forget the temporary nature of everything. At times like this, it's often a good tactic to reflect on the impermanence of everything. Even just saying out loud "this is impermanent" can help. Well, it's a lot better than swearing at the top of your lungs! Things like boring paperwork, being on hold in an automated phone queue or stuck in a traffic jam are some examples. I mean, all you need to do is think of a mundane task that drives you nuts and you'll have a good example. For me, cleaning the bathroom and food shopping would make my list. But, all of these things are impermanent. And we need to remember this when we get frustrated by them.

I find that the concept of impermanence can also be helpful when dealing with difficult and uncomfortable situations (think pain and powerful emotions). Knowing that the situation will change or pass can help us to accept what we are dealing with and remember that it's not permanent.

So, the moral of the story: embrace change! It's going to happen whether you like it or not. Quit complaining, roll with the punches and know that nothing lasts forever.

CONNECTING WITH NATURE

One of my favourite things to do that helps to invoke a strong sense of *sympatheia*, is to go out and connect with nature. I am acutely aware that being immersed in nature affects my mental health in an extremely positive way. I also feel more connected to my environment and the world in general. If I spend an entire day on the computer and don't leave the house to get some air, I feel rough.

Some of the most profound and moving experiences of my life have taken place in nature. An example of this is when I visited the Grand Canyon during my period of peak anxiety. At the time, I was a complete mess and my anxiety was out of control. Just getting to the canyon was an ordeal. The drive had freaked me out and I was in a terrible place mentally. However, as soon as we parked the car and I saw the canyon, my mind settled. It was such an awe-inspiring environment that I instantly felt at peace. It was a real sense of deep calm and connection that is hard to put into words. The depth and vastness of the canyon completely blew me away. Awe is the only word that I think does it justice – although even that feels like an inferior word. The interesting thing is that as soon as we left the canyon, I felt horrific again. This slice of nature was so powerful that it completely disrupted my peak anxiety.

There's a philosophical concept called The Sublime, which I also find fascinating (not from Stoicism but really interesting). The Sublime in nature refers to how the power of the natural world can make us feel vulnerable yet inspired and connected at the same time – an awe-inducing vista that also has the potential to destroy us can create this feeling. Imagine a giant chasm/a huge mountain range/sprawling canyons/epic sea cliffs/barren deserts/frozen arctic icescapes ... All of these environments are truly beautiful but equally dangerous. Visiting them can have a profound shift on our minds. They can make us feel small and insignificant yet still inspire us because they are so overwhelmingly beautiful.

I think this is why I love outdoor sports so much. Activities like wild swimming, trail running and mountaineering allow me to connect with nature in an engaging way. They make me feel alive. The thing is, we don't have to travel far to feel this – simply making space for nature in our lives can do this. It also doesn't have to be anywhere epic and remote – any slice of nature will do the job!

There's another interesting concept that ties in with all of this called *ecopsychology*. This field of study explores the importance of connecting with nature from a psychological perspective. Basically, it concludes that spending time in nature is key to living a good life. The Japanese have a therapy called *shinrin-yoku* – meaning "forest bathing". Participants are encouraged to spend time among the trees and connect with the great outdoors. This is pretty much ecopsychology in action.

Another thing that can be great for developing a deeper sense of connection with the world around us is to learn more about the natural world. For me, I can't watch enough nature documentaries (David Attenborough programmes are a personal favourite of mine). There's nothing quite like learning about weird and wonderful creatures as a way to feel inspired by the natural world. Just read about a hairy-chested yeti crab or the mites that live on your eyelashes and you'll get what I mean. Yes – there are crabs that have hairy chests! And yes, that's also right – you have little mites living on your eyelashes. They are a third of a millimetre long, translucent and feast on dead skin and oil. Yummy. Nature is truly incredible.

If we learn about nature and spend time actively engaging with it, we are more likely to look after it. Nature is all we have – it's what we are! We are all connected and share this planet together. The Stoic view of *sympatheia* can help us to remember this.

BEN'S MIND-BOGGLING FACTS

By contemplating mind-boggling facts, our brains can feel overwhelmed. It's this sense of crushing awe that can be interesting to reflect on. We are all part of this universe and spending time thinking about big and small concepts can help us to feel connected to everything in an interesting way. I love learning crazy stats that make my brain spin. I've compiled a little list below to get you thinking. Spend a bit of time reflecting on these facts:

1. There are approximately 360,000 births every day. That's four a second.
2. There are approximately 150,000 deaths every day. That's nearly two every second.
3. There are approximately 1,000,000,000,000,000,000,000,000 (1 septillion) stars in the observable universe ... That's only the bit we can see, though. That number is mad. This is similar to the number of grains of sand on planet Earth. (Imagine all of the beaches and deserts on the planet. That's a lot of sand.)
4. There are approximately 7,000,000,000,000,000,000,000,000,000,000 (7 octillion) atoms in a human body. This is similar to the number of times I ate pizza during lockdown in 2020.
5. Atoms are mostly empty space. You are therefore made up of over 99% nothingness ...
6. The human body is about 60% water. So, based on the last two facts, humanity is like a very empty glass of water.
7. Approximately five billion pizzas are sold worldwide each year.
8. Bees can be used to detect bombs ... OK – maybe we're drifting off a little here.
9. The average human heart beats more than 2.5 billion times in an average life.
10. If you were to compress the history of the universe into a calendar year, all of human history would only take up the last minute. So essentially, an entire year and then at 11:59pm on December 31 – we appear. How small and short our existence is in the cosmic scale of things.

FINAL THOUGHTS

The Stoics didn't contemplate things from a cosmic perspective as a way to feel depressed about how fleeting life was. This concept was used to feel grateful for the incredibly precious gift of life. It was also used to detach from the intensity of tough moments by highlighting how cosmically small their grumbles were.

Thinking about the big picture gives us perspective which can be liberating – there's a real lightness that comes from not being so caught up in the minutia of the day. There's also a lightness that comes from feeling connected to nature and humanity. The Stoics were really onto something with this!

We are lucky to be alive. We should embrace what we have and live for now – because nothing else exists. Enjoy your cheese and pickle sandwich. Be grateful. It will all pass anyway.

*"Meditate often on the interconnectedness
and mutual interdependence of all things
in the universe. For in a sense, all things are
mutually woven together and therefore have
an affinity for each other – for one thing follows
after another according to their tension of
movement, their sympathetic stirrings, and the
unity of all substance."*

Marcus Aurelius

PRACTICAL EXERCISES

The purpose of these exercises is to make us feel connected with the world around us and instil a greater sense of awe for life.

THE COSMIC VIEW/VIEW FROM ABOVE

Spend some time looking at images of the Earth from space. There are so many out there to flick through so this should keep you busy for a while. Look at the beauty of our planet as a whole and contemplate your part in its preservation.

Chris Hadfield has some fantastic footage from his time spent on the ISS (International Space Station), so be sure to check out his content.

Also have a go at completing the *View from Above* exercise mentioned earlier in the principle. It's not a bad way to get some perspective!

CONNECTING WITH NATURE

Search up the natural wonders near to you and pay them a visit. While there, sit quietly and spend time contemplating your part in nature. Reflecting on the cosmic perspective of everything is a very Stoic exercise indeed. Time in nature can be a great way of connecting with this concept.

IMPERMANENCE

Find some old photos and observe how much you have changed. Be glad that your hair doesn't still look like that! Now, think about how quickly life is flying by and expand this to contemplate the impermanence of everything.

Try to apply the concept of impermanence to the things you face in daily life. Think about how cosmically small that traffic jam is … Think about how universally insignificant that queue at the supermarket was … All things pass. Remember this. Use your journal to make notes on your experiences.

FINDING NEMO'S WEIRD COUSIN

Exploring the weird and wonderful creatures on Earth can help us to feel more connected to our planet. Google a blobfish or watch a nature documentary to encounter a wide range of incredibly diverse life. By appreciating nature, we can respect it and care for it more. Connecting with science and nature can help us to feel like a part of it. Here are some of the most unusual creatures I've come across that you should definitely check out:

- Blobfish
- Giant Isopod
- Hairy-chested Yeti Crab
- Axolotl
- Sea Pigs

MIND-BOGGLING FACTS

In the style of my mind-boggling facts section, start your own collection of facts that make you feel both inspired and humbled. Space is a great topic. The microscopic world is a great topic. Time is a great topic. You have plenty of options, so start exploring!

Collect your mind-bogglers in one place (maybe on your phone or in your journal) and keep adding to the list over time. Come and share them with me on social media too – I can't get enough of them!

JOURNALING PROMPTS

Your journaling exercise for this principle is twofold:

Firstly, start collecting all of your mind-boggling stats and weird creatures. You should also list your local natural wonders and use the journal as a place to track how many you have visited. Maybe create a nature-based bucket list. There are so many things that you could add to this list – different environments, unfamiliar types of plants and trees, a cross-section of wildlife. You are literally spoilt for choice with this.

Secondly, write about your experience of connecting with nature and viewing the world from above. Did you feel different in nature when you started to expand your perspective of everything and think about your part in it? What did it feel like when you were exploring space from your phone/computer? Did it make you feel small? Or connected? Or both?

PART 3

PUTTING STOICISM INTO PRACTICE

Well, that's a lot of philosophy I've just thrown at you! Ten big ideas. Fifty practical exercises. And if you count The Stoic Golden Rule and The Cardinal Virtues mentioned near the start of the book, you have even more ideas to work with.

This is a lot of information to process and the thing is, it's easy to forget all of this if you don't use it. These ideas will quickly fade from the memory if you don't actively engage with them. That would be a shame, so in this section of the book I'm going to outline the best way for you to be proactive and bring all of these ideas together and start thinking like a Stoic. There are so many ways to do this and you can have a lot of fun in the process.

13

STOIC WORDS

A great way to consolidate all of your Stoic knowledge is to collect your favourite Stoic quotes. Choose lines that represent key ideas and that make complete sense to you. There's no specific list for you to follow but learning a few quotes off by heart that you like can be incredibly handy. Whipping them out when you're dealing with a setback or challenging situation can help keep Stoicism in the forefront of your mind.

I'm not saying that you need to recite these quotes in a Shakespearean manner at the top of your voice. What I'm suggesting is that you have a series of quotes that you can visualize in your mind's eye at times of need. The more you do this, the quicker they will come to you when facing difficulty. Essentially, you're programming your mind to remind you of this ancient wisdom. Here are some of my favourites:

"When someone is properly grounded in life, they shouldn't have to look outside themselves for approval."

Epictetus

"Be tolerant with others and strict with yourself."

Marcus Aurelius

*"True happiness is to enjoy the present,
without anxious dependence upon the future."*

Seneca

*"You will earn the respect of all if you begin by
earning the respect of yourself."*

Musonius Rufus

*"Wellbeing is realized by small steps, but is
truly no small thing."*

Zeno

*"The happiness of your life depends upon the
quality of your thoughts."*

Marcus Aurelius

*"No person has the power to have everything
they want, but it is in their power not to want
what they don't have, and to cheerfully put to
good use what they do have."*

Seneca

Pick quotes that you like and record them in your journal or keep them on your phone. Why not print them out or write them down and place them in different parts of the house? How about the bathroom mirror? Or on your fridge? Or the front of your cereal box? Having these words in your mind can be a wonderful way to contemplate and embed ideas.

Some people have taken this further and have Stoic quotes tattooed on their bodies. *Disclaimer – I'm not encouraging you to get Stoic tattoos all over your body (that's your choice). I just want to point out how important these words can be to lots of people. The quotes can be powerful and many Stoics want them close by.

STOIC MAXIMS

Maxims are concise and easily memorable rules. They encapsulate ideas effectively in short sentences and can help us to keep these ideas in our minds. Creating our own maxims that reflect Stoic concepts is another fantastic way to keep the philosophy close to heart.

I have a series of Stoic maxims that I like to say to myself when facing difficult situations. These are the three that I regularly use (particularly if I'm having to deal with a setback):

1. This is character-building
2. Focus on what you CAN control
3. This will pass

These three simple maxims help me to focus on the following Stoic concepts: The Cardinal Virtues, The Stoic Golden Rule and Impermanence. These concepts are great for dealing with tough situations for three reasons:

1. They help me to give value to the situation I am facing by giving me the chance to build character and ensure that I am dealing with the problem Stoically.
2. They help me to put my head in the right place – by focusing on what I can actually do about the problem (what I can control).

3. They help me to see the bigger picture and remember that this problem will eventually pass.

It's quick to recite these maxims and I don't have to do it out loud. Although sometimes I do! It's an unbelievably effective way to get my mindset into the right place.

If the problem or setback is particularly tricky, I work through each of the maxims in more detail and expand the dialogue. I can use logic to drill down on each of these points to ground myself in the middle of a crisis.

Feel free to modify these maxims or use different ones – be creative and come up with concise summaries of the Stoic ideas that are most relevant to you. Remember that something short tends to work well as it's easier to remember. It also doesn't take a long time to recite and gets to the point quicker. Double bonus!

READING THE STOICS

Along with testing out the ideas in this book in the real world, I'd like to encourage you to read the Stoics.

Reading the ancient texts is an important part of thinking like a Stoic. You've already encountered a lot of their words in these pages as I've been quoting them left, right and centre, but reading their full works is where it's at. If this book has inspired you to check out the original Stoics, I will feel like it has been a success. Their work is brilliant!

I write about how to build a Stoic library at the end of the book, so we will revisit this theme in detail then. But before we get to that, I want to introduce you to the Stoic Challenges.

14

THE STOIC CHALLENGES

Alright, let's have some fun. I've created a few Stoic Challenges to help you explore different ways to bring Stoicism into your daily life. They range in difficulty and length but all share the same goal – to help you consolidate the ideas in this book and put them into practice. Have a look through them and see which appeals to you the most. By selecting and committing to one of the following programmes, you will take everything you've learned so far and go deeper into Stoic philosophy in a practical way. Exciting times!

My suggested Stoic Challenges are:

1. The 10-Day Stoic Challenge
2. The Month-Long Stoic Challenge
3. The Year-Long Stoic Challenge
4. Ben's Stoic Challenge Day

I'll explain each one and you can then decide which is the best option for you.

THE 10-DAY STOIC CHALLENGE

Goal: The goal with this challenge is to give you a practical flavour of each principle in this book, plus to establish some

Stoic routines and embark on reading some original Stoic writing every day.

Time Required: 30 minutes a day, for 10 days.

Why: This is a great way to start testing out and experiencing the ideas in this book without it feeling overwhelming. The 10 days will give you enough time to get an appreciation of Stoicism in action. It's a nice and easy way to get your foot in the Stoic door.

What You Will Need to Complete the Challenge:
- Access to the Internet
- *Meditations* by Marcus Aurelius
- Notepad or journal
- Resources for the practical exercises you end up selecting

Task List:
- Read *Meditations* by Marcus Aurelius
- Complete one practical exercise from each principle (1 per day for 10 days)
- Establish a morning and/or evening routine for Stoic exercises and reading
- Journal every evening
- Learn three Stoic quotes off by heart
- Keep The Stoic Golden Rule in mind throughout the 10-day period (as much as possible)

How: This challenge won't take up loads of your time but you will need to get a little organized. Firstly, you'll need to carve out some time at the start and end of the day so that you can read, reflect and complete your chosen challenge.

I'd recommend kicking off each day with some time spent reading *Meditations* by Aurelius. After this, pick a challenge for that day (one per day – each from one of the ten principles) and think about how to incorporate it into your routine.

At the end of the day, spend some time journaling and reflecting on everything that happened to you since waking up. Write about the lessons learned and the things you were grateful for. You could also follow Epictetus' example and write about the good, the bad and what's left to be done. You have plenty of options.

THE MONTH-LONG STOIC CHALLENGE

Goal: This challenge will give you a solid understanding of each principle in this book over a longer period. You will read three of the most important books in Stoic philosophy and also establish a morning/evening routine while testing out Stoic journaling along the way.

Time Required: 1 month (30 minutes to an hour a day)

Why: This is the perfect way to give Stoicism a full test drive. A month is a relatively short space of time but you can achieve a lot if you are disciplined. You will get a real sense of what ideas from Stoicism work for you with this challenge. This is a great way to bring the philosophy to life.

What You Will Need to Complete the Challenge:

- Access to the Internet
- *Meditations* by Marcus Aurelius
- *Discourses and Selected Writings* by Epictetus
- *Letters from a Stoic* by Seneca
- Notepad or journal
- Relevant resources for the practical exercises you end up selecting

Task List:

- Read *Meditations* by Marcus Aurelius
- Read *Discourses and Selected Writings* by Epictetus

- Read *Letters from a Stoic* by Seneca
- Complete two practical exercises from each principle (20 exercises over the month)
- Establish a morning and/or evening routine for Stoic exercises and reading
- Journal every single evening (use the journaling prompts from the principles to help)
- Learn 10 Stoic quotes off by heart
- Keep The Stoic Golden Rule in mind throughout the month (as much as possible)
- Keep The Cardinal Virtues in mind throughout the month (as much as possible)

How: The reading task for this challenge will take up quite a bit of time so give yourself enough space to work through the recommended books. Alongside your reading, make sure that you establish a journaling habit in the evening and give yourself plenty of time to complete practical exercises from each principle. Revisit the journaling prompts from each principle for inspiration. You should complete two exercises from each principle across the month (20 in total). The goal is to have a lot of fun with this so choose exercises that you really like the sound of and plan your time accordingly.

THE YEAR-LONG STOIC CHALLENGE

Goal: This challenge involves more commitment than the others but will help you to establish a very deep and detailed understanding of Stoicism.
Time Required: 1 Year/Ongoing
Why: If you work through all of the tasks in this challenge, you will have a better understanding of Stoic philosophy than the majority of the people on this planet. You will have read many

of the core texts, have a thorough understanding of the history and will have put the ideas into practice. It has the potential to completely change the way you view the world. Not too shabby!

What You Will Need to Complete the Challenge:
- Access to the Internet
- All the books mentioned in the *How to Build a Stoic Library* section at the end of this book
- Notepad or journal
- Relevant resources for all practical exercises in this book

Task List:
- Complete every single practical exercise in this book (50 in total)
- Read everything on the *How to Build a Stoic Library* list
- Establish a morning and/or evening routine for Stoic exercises and reading
- Establish a journaling habit that has stuck (use the journaling prompts from the principles and Epictetus' self-reflecting evening routine)
- Learn multiple Stoic quotes off by heart
- Engage with the Stoic community
- Listen to interviews or podcasts with prominent Stoic thinkers

How: There are several tasks for you to work through in order to complete this challenge. However, the two big ones are making your way through the reading list, and completing all of the practical exercises from this book. There are many ways that you can tackle this and you should decide how you plan your time. But, for the sake of getting your organizational juices flowing, here is a potential structure you might like to follow:

Each month work through all of the exercises from one of the principles in this book and read one of the book recommendations. For example, in Month 1 – work through all of the practical exercises in the Voluntary Discomfort principle and read *Meditations* by Aurelius. In Month 2 – work through all of the practical exercises in the Perception principle and read *Discourses and Selected Writings* by Epictetus … You get the idea.

By doing things this way, it means you only have one Stoic book a month to read and approximately one practical exercise a week to try. Easy! You might want to mix up the principles and jumble up the practical exercises to keep things fresh, but that's entirely up to you.

Along with the practical exercises and the large reading list, establishing a journaling habit and a little morning and/or evening routine is also on the agenda. Committing to this might be tricky so don't feel disheartened if you occasionally drop the habit and have to re-establish it. We're looking for long-term change here and that means that sometimes life will get in the way and your habits and routines might get broken – but it's what happens next that is important. Are you able to pick things up again and carry on?

I'd also encourage you to start engaging with the Stoic community. Spend time watching videos about Stoicism on YouTube. Listen to podcasts and interviews with modern Stoic thinkers and writers. Read articles on www.modernstoicism.com and get busy immersing yourself in these ancient ideas.

Consider how this could slot into your life on a long-term basis. How would you complete these tasks across a year? Although this is a lot of stuff to work through, you do have a year to do it. The workload isn't too intense and I believe that Project Stoic could comfortably be incorporated into a busy life.

BEN'S STOIC CHALLENGE DAY

Goal: The goal with this challenge is to spend a whole day living like an extreme Stoic.

Time Required: 24 hours

Why: If you want the ultimate crash course in Stoicism, this is it. All you need is 24 hours and you can get a real sense of some core Stoic themes. Granted, this is a bit of a crazy way to do things and it will require a lot of effort on your part – but that's all part of the fun and what you were looking for, right?

If you complete my Stoic Challenge Day, I'm confident it'll be a day that you won't soon forget.

What You Will Need to Complete the Challenge:
- Access to the Internet
- A banana
- Some string
- *Meditations* by Marcus Aurelius
- Notepad or journal

Task List:
- Sleep on the floor without a pillow or mattress (page 35)
- Take a cold shower (page 34)
- Only drink water (page 42)
- Only eat simple food – and avoid sugar (page 42)
- Complete a pet banana/vegetable walk in a busy public space (page 36)
- Read *Meditations* by Marcus Aurelius
- Spend 10 minutes on the *memento mori* death meditation (page 143)
- Spend 10 minutes on the negative visualization exercises (page 108)
- Listen to *The Olatunji Concert: The Last Live Recording* by John Coltrane (page 53)
- Spend one hour in mini-exile paying attention to the mind (page 56)
- Complete the "debate time" exercise without losing control of the situation (page 138)

- Establish a list of role models (page 95)
- Establish a list of anti-role models (page 96)
- Complete three random acts of kindness (page 136)
- Watch mind-boggling space videos on YouTube (page 166)
- Read some articles on www.modernstoicism.com
- Learn three Stoic quotes off by heart
- Create a *memento mori* reminder (skeleton/skull picture, etc.) (page 150)
- Complete a demanding workout (page 42)
- Reflect on the day in the evening by journaling on events and lessons

How: This entire day is all about Stoicism. From the moment you wake up to the moment you go to sleep, you will be welcoming Stoic philosophy into your life. So, let's run through what you need to do …

There are 20 Stoic tasks for you to work through in order to complete this challenge. The goal is to get through all of them within a 24-hour period. This won't be easy … But that's the point. It's a great way to push yourself with a few of the ideas from this book.

You will need to organize your time accordingly, so I suggest looking through the list and deciding what order you're going to tackle everything. There is no strict structure for this, so grab a pen and some paper and start planning your day.

Note that certain tasks will last all day (only drink water/ eat simple food), some will take a while (read *Meditations* by Marcus Aurelius) and some will be over in a flash (cold shower/ banana walk). You might want to load the front half of the day with the shorter tasks and then settle into some reading and reflection later in the day. Or not. There are so many ways that you can complete the day so have fun and be creative with the way you organize your time.

It would be a nice idea to document your day with photos or a short video. If you do this, why not share your experience with others on social media? Come and say hi online if you do – my Instagram handle is @dothingsthatchallengyou and my Twitter account is @iambenaldridge.

Alternatively, a detailed journal entry for the day will not only mark off one of the tasks, but it will also help you to have a well-documented reminder of all the crazy things you ended up doing in 24 hours.

Completing this Stoic Challenge Day with friends and family might also be a nice way of sharing the day and introducing others to some Stoic principles at the same time.

Good luck with this one; it'll be a quirky day if you go for it!

So, there you have it – four challenges that you can get stuck into. Each one is likely to appeal to different people, but I feel that all of them have the potential to help you deepen your understanding of Stoic philosophy.

15

THE FUTURE OF STOICISM

Let's be honest, life doesn't look like it's suddenly going to get any easier – we have many issues that we will need to work on together to resolve, manage and prepare for. From social injustices and climate change to the introduction of Artificial Intelligence, humanity is going to need to address these issues in a proactive way if we want to progress as a civilization. If only there was some type of philosophical guidance that could help us to navigate all of this uncertainty ...

I believe that Stoicism offers us a structure for a lot of these future challenges. Whether as individuals or as a society, the Stoic way of seeing the world can help us to bring objectivity and fairness to these issues. The fact that Stoic philosophy is heavily based on reasoning and logic means that it complements science and progression in the 21st century well. This is a real positive and something that makes Stoicism future-proof in my eyes. Logic and reasoning are the bedrock to Stoic thought. Without them, things can start to get messy and unscientific. Reason and logic are able to change their minds if new facts come along and update the dialogue. This quality alone is one of the most important things we need in modern life – the ability to change our opinions on things as our understanding develops. Reason and logic don't encourage us to stubbornly hold on to opinions that aren't benefitting anyone.

Something that you will hear a lot about from the Stoics is the idea of "living in agreement with nature". The Stoics believed that to live in accordance with nature was to use the rational component of our minds. This was seen as a gift. The ability to reason helps us to thrive. If we don't use reason and just revert back to living like a bunch of wild animals, we won't be fulfilling our human obligations. What better way to face the future than with clear thinking and sound logic?

As a philosophy, Stoicism is open to progression. It's not a fixed set of ideas that must be rigidly followed – these concepts can move forward and evolve with us. We live in a dynamic universe and it's important for our ideas to be able to grow as our understanding of science and the universe changes. Robert Dobbin, the Stoic translator and editor acknowledges this at the start of his Penguin Classics translation of Epictetus' *Discourses and Selected Writings*:

"Indeed, the Stoics' openness to revision was a particular strength of their school."

Robert Dobbin

I'm incredibly excited about the future of Stoicism as we see it rise in popularity. I believe that this Stoic resurgence, or Stoic revolution (if you're an optimist), has come at the right time. This philosophy can help to bring humans together. It doesn't matter what your background is or if you have a religion in your life – Stoicism can be a framework for life and connect people from all over the planet. It can help us to come together and address big global issues with the right attitude. Yes, I'm an idealist, but we've got to start somewhere!

I think the wave is building and we will soon see Stoicism moving into the mainstream. Well, I certainly hope so. This would be a good thing for humanity. I'm excited to be a part of this movement, and by you engaging with these ideas, you are part of this too!

STOICISM IN SCHOOLS

Stoic philosophy would be an incredible addition to the school system – I see a gap waiting to be filled. If these ideas were taught to the younger generation, it would have a hugely positive impact on their mental wellbeing and ability to handle adversity.

I've actually worked in education for well over a decade now so I guess that's why I'm so passionate about bringing these ideas to younger people. I've predominately worked in primary schools but also have experience in secondary schools and up to age 18. Stoicism would benefit all of these age groups in a host of ways.

I'm keen to pass on this philosophy as it was something I was never exposed to as a kid. When I was young, the school system missed out some hugely important life-essentials. Mental health – mental what? How to manage your emotions – just get on with it! What to do when things go wrong – you failed, here's your grade ... I learned how to calculate pi, something which I have literally never used since leaving school, but didn't understand how to deal with strong emotions, manage my mental health or understand the best way to deal with failures and setbacks. I felt like the education system had failed me. I know that things are changing these days but life skills are incredibly important – and Stoic philosophy has many to offer.

It would also be a highly engaging and practical subject. As you've seen with a lot of the challenges in this book, there are practical ways to bring these ancient concepts to life. If you get a teenager to walk a pet banana through a busy public space, they're going to remember that experience for a long time!

Novelty things stick with us. I remember melting jelly babies in a science class. This learning experience was a beacon of hope for me among a bland syllabus that left me uninspired. Stoic ideas could be taught in a fun, crazy, engaging, practical, inspiring and infinitely helpful manner to the next generation –

who will all have to face their own set of unique challenges and adversity. Being a young adult can be tough. It's a formative time as we are starting to learn more about who we really are.

The other great thing about introducing Stoicism to schools is that you could also sneak in a bit of history along the way – what better way to learn about the Romans and the Greeks than by using their concepts in modern life?! Two boxes ticked!

From a young age these Stoic ideas can help our children and the next generation to develop the resilience to deal with life's ups and downs. These concepts could be part of their toolkit for dealing with modern life. Personally, I'd encourage a practical approach by getting them to test out these ideas in the real world. As they get older, actually reading the Stoics would be a good way to deepen their understanding. So, Epictetus on the school curriculum ... Yes please!

MY GRAND STOIC VISION

I have a dream ... Well, it's an optimistic view of where all of this could go. Firstly, I'd like to see more Stoic events taking place in local communities. There are some fantastic events already happening and this is mainly down to the team at www.modernstoicism.com – they are doing an incredible job of putting on Stoic events and encouraging others to do the same. For example, Stoicon is a week-long Stoic convention that attracts international speakers from across the globe and thousands of attendees. There are also Stoicon-x events – similar to TEDx events – locally run gatherings that anyone can put on (yes, you could bring one of these events to your local town). But, I'm greedy ... I want this to expand even more.

Wouldn't it be great to have buildings dedicated to Stoicism where people can gather and discuss these ideas?! I know this sounds a bit religious – but I think it can still retain a secular feel. Having set buildings (or even a giant porch – like the *Stoa Poikile*) would be great for developing a local community of Stoics. So, who's up for building this? Anyone?

I'd also love to see more Stoicism in modern culture – art, literature, movies and music. A few blockbuster movies would certainly help put these ideas on the map. Just imagine Sylvester Stallone playing Epictetus … Yes, that's a wonderful image.

So, to conclude – think about what has happened with the mindfulness and meditation movement over the last few years. We have a huge amount of resources for these ideas and science is confirming why we should use them in modern life. I would love Stoicism to be in a similar place to this. And from there, who knows where it will go.

16

UPGRADING STOICISM

When we encounter new ideas, I believe there's value in considering how we would improve upon or further develop them. This gets us to look at the limits of the idea and contemplate an upgrade. This is how the BBQ-base pizza was created!

The same is true for philosophy. After we've got to know the core ideas well, we can contemplate what works for us and what doesn't. We can think about what tweaks we would like to make, and we can apply them. We then ask: would this improve the idea? If it does, fantastic. If not, it's back to the drawing board. This is critical thinking in action.

Stoicism is a wonderful and comprehensive philosophy with a great set of ideas that work remarkably well in the modern era. There aren't actually loads of alterations I would make to it. Granted, I'm not that into the Zeusy-ness of the ancients, but if we view Zeus as synonymous with nature, we don't have to get caught up with the talk of an archaic god. That works for me!

I know, I know – who am I to sit here yakking on about altering a philosophy that is thousands of years old and works perfectly well. But at this point it's important to remember Seneca's wise words:

"I do not bind myself to some particular one of the Stoic masters; I, too, have the right to form an opinion."

Seneca

How would I upgrade Stoicism? What would I do? Well, I would suggest two contributions to the philosophy. These are two small developments of Stoic thought that, in my opinion, would work well. They aren't alterations – they are simple additions:

1. Meditation
2. The Anti-Bucket List

MEDITATION

In Stoic philosophy, traditional meditation isn't really a thing. I would like to suggest that it becomes a thing. Sitting down quietly and focusing on settling the mind by breathing would be a wonderful practice as part of a daily Stoic routine.

Being present and conscious of the moment is something that the Stoics talk about. They even had a word for it – *Prosochê*. This essentially means mindfulness – the ability to be present and not caught up in thoughts. OK, the actual translation is "attention", and it's a little different to the mindfulness we know in the modern world, but having a presence of mind is important and a theme I'd like to build on. Seneca puts it eloquently:

"The whole future lies in uncertainty: live immediately."

Seneca

As the concept of being present isn't a new one in Stoic philosophy, training this skill is a perfectly reasonable suggestion. And the best way to actually train this skill is through meditation practice. Science tells us that the more we meditate, the better we become at being present. The process actually alters the grey matter in our brains by stimulating different parts of it. This helps us to increase our attention span, which is something that is extremely important in modern life. We are bombarded with pings, beeps and rings from our smartphones and electronic devices and information overload can be a serious problem. We suffer mental fatigue and our brains crave stimulation. Meditation counters this. It gives us space to think; it helps us to be present and to value what we have in life. As you can guess, I'm a big fan.

Meditation helps us to live in the moment and it also helps us to build gratitude. It allows us to understand our minds and perceptions better, and to *not* believe everything we think (something very handy if you have a negative internal dialogue). It also pushes us to relax and de-stress. Seriously, if you aren't meditating, why not? You could even combine it with some of the Stoic practices mentioned in this book.

A quick note – the Stoics do already have a meditation practice but it's more contemplative and reflective. It tends to focus on self-reflection and thought experiments – journaling being one of the key ways that they would do this. Negative visualization and *memento mori* are two more examples.

If you fancy giving traditional meditation a go, here is a very quick rundown of the process:

1. Set a timer for 10 minutes
2. Sit somewhere comfortable where you won't be distracted
3. Focus on your breath – in and out
4. Repeat until the timer rings

Easy! Well, not always. You will likely get distracted and forget to focus on your breathing but this is normal, so don't beat yourself up about it. Simply keep bringing your attention back to your breath each time you are distracted. It requires a little discipline to get into a regular routine but the benefits and rewards are worth the effort.

Guided meditations work really well too. My favourite apps are *Waking Up* by Sam Harris and *Headspace*. You can't go wrong with either of these.

THE ANTI-BUCKET LIST

My second contribution to Stoicism would be the anti-bucket list. I wrote about how I started using this in my life earlier in the book. The idea is simple – you create a list of things that scare you (and that you don't really want to do), and then actively seek them out. If you've worked through any of the practical exercises in this book, you may have already started creating your list. It can be a revealing process!

When I talk about my journey with voluntary discomfort, the anti-bucket list tends to get a lot of attention. And I think it should. It feels counter-intuitive and people can really visualize the process of challenging their personal fears. As mentioned earlier, fear and play don't normally go together, so it's an intriguing proposition – to play with your fears. It sounds bizarre but it's an idea that a lot of people enjoy and have connected with.

It would be a great addition to Stoic philosophy as it's essentially an extension of voluntary discomfort but specifically for things that we fear. By seeking out ideas that scare us, we get the opportunity to practise adversity – and this, in essence, is what voluntary discomfort is all about.

So, those are my two additions. If I could help progress Stoic philosophy, this is what I would add. They take Stoic ideas a little further and are more extensions of ideas, rather than introducing something new and radical.

Have a think about the ideas you have encountered in this book and consider which ones you have connected with. Would you upgrade any of them? Or would you like to keep Stoicism as it is? Food for thought.

I personally love the idea of combining philosophical concepts, so am always on the lookout for new ideas. Being open is the key.

FINAL THOUGHTS

Stoic philosophy has had a profound impact on my life – after all, I have written an entire book about it! I've done my best to share Stoicism in a light and accessible way and I really hope that some of the principles and ideas in this book have resonated with you. They can be life-changing if implemented and I feel lucky to be able to share them with you.

Writing about the Stoics has helped me to further my understanding of the philosophy and I continue to be impressed by this timeless wisdom. I always try to apply anything new that I've learned in a practical way and love coming up with challenges to test out concepts. From banana walks to mini self-exiles, I have had a lot of fun putting Stoicism to the test in the real world and this is something I will continue to do. So, watch this space!

Although I got into Stoicism because I needed a way to build resilience, I have come to realize how much more than this the philosophy offers. There are concepts here that map wonderfully onto modern life and can guide us in countless situations. It's rich and nuanced and is something that I now use as a framework for how to live. I truly believe that this philosophy can change humanity for the better. It encourages us to look at our characters and ensure that as individuals we are taking responsibility for our behaviour. It encourages us to develop a forgiving attitude toward those around us and to cultivate a deeper appreciation for life itself. It inspires us to connect with nature and with others in a meaningful way. If we all think like Stoics a little more, I'm hopeful that the world will be a better place.

So, take some time to appreciate the beauty around you. Stop to smell the roses. Remember that this life will one day end and you will not be able to eat pizza anymore. Remember that you will continue to face uncertainty. And that you have little control over what happens to you. But this is alright. You have the strength in you to face any challenge – and you can certainly train yourself to be better at doing this. Focus on your response to external events and focus on your character. This is how you find some semblance of control in a chaotic and uncontrollable world. This is how you build a resilient and fulfilling life and bring ancient philosophy to the modern world.

I wish you the best of luck!

"How long are you going to wait before you demand the best for yourself?"

Epictetus

HOW TO BUILD A STOIC LIBRARY

Reading the Stoics is an essential part of understanding the philosophy in more detail. You can't beat hearing it from the horse's mouth, so it makes sense for you to actually dive into these ancient texts.

I've included a comprehensive list of books to give you a solid and deep understanding of their ideas. Feel free to pick and choose from this list, but I advise heading to the actual Stoics first.

Please note: There are many different translations of the Stoics' works, so for the sake of keeping things simple, I've included my favourite translations in this reading list. **Please also note:** A lot of the quotes in this book come from a variety of sources. The books mentioned in this section have been integral to gathering them.

THE STOICS

Aurelius, Marcus. *Meditations.* (Gregory Hay's translation) Weidenfeld and Nicholson, 2004
This is one of the most important Stoic texts and arguably one of the most important philosophical books of all time. It's a great place to start. Plus, I've been yakking on about Aurelius for a long time now so you should definitely check him out!

Epictetus. *Discourses and Selected Writings.*
Penguin Classics, 2008
This is a collection of short books that are essentially ancient blog posts on a variety of different topics. *The Enchiridion* – which is a short guide for living well – is included in this edition (although you can pick up a copy of this separately). Both are great reads and packed with timeless wisdom.

Seneca. *Letters from a Stoic.* Penguin Classics, 2004
This is a collection of letters that Seneca wrote to his friend, Lucilius. Tons of topics are covered and Seneca offers plenty of great life advice that's still relevant to this very day. I think of Seneca as a Roman "Oprah", and this book really helps to consolidate that image in my mind.

Seneca. *On the Shortness of Life.* Penguin, 2004
This book does what it says on the tin: it's all about how brief life is and why we shouldn't waste it. It's also a quick read, so a great way to get a flavour of Seneca.

Rufus, Musonius. *That One Should Disdain Hardships: The Teachings of a Roman Stoic.* Yale University Press, 2020
This is a series of short essays that explore the Stoicism of Rufus. There's also a nice collection of his quotes and sayings at the end of the book. It's a short read but covers many wide-ranging topics. I highly recommend it.

ABOUT THE STOICS

There are a lot of books on Stoicism out there, and it's easy to become overwhelmed. However, the following writers are doing an incredible job of spreading the wisdom of the Stoics in the modern world. These are hands down my favourite books about Stoicism. They are all very accessible and do a wonderful job of exploring these ancient ideas.

Hanselman, Stephen and Holiday, Ryan. *The Daily Stoic*. Profile Books, 2016

Every day for an entire year you get a Stoic quote and a brief exploration of the quote. This is a fantastic book to introduce into your Stoic routine – just read one quote in the morning and ponder it for the rest of the day. Perfect!

Hanselman, Stephen and Holiday, Ryan. *Lives of the Stoics*. Profile Books, 2020

This book gives a detailed history of all the major Stoics. It also explores those that aren't well known. It's a wonderful resource for those interested in the history of the Stoics and the origins of Stoicism.

Robertson, Donald. *How to Think Like a Roman Emperor*. Griffin, 2020

This book is an exploration of Marcus Aurelius' life and approach to Stoic philosophy. It's a brilliant read and a great way to get to know more about the most famous Stoic of all time.

Robertson, Donald. *Stoicism and the Art of Happiness*. Teach Yourself, 2018

My other recommendation from Donald Robertson is this detailed and comprehensive look at the philosophy in general.

It's superb. Combining his knowledge of modern therapy (he is a practising therapist) and ancient history, you're in safe hands here.

Pigliucci, Massimo. *How to Be a Stoic: Ancient Wisdom for Modern Living.* **Rider, 2017**
This is a great book for developing a broad understanding of Stoic philosophy. It looks in detail at key themes and explains them in a clean, crisp and precise manner. Perfect for getting your head around complex topics.

Pigliucci, Massimo. *The Stoic Guide to a Happy Life: 53 Brief Lessons for Living.* **Rider, 2020**
Massimo has updated Epictetus' *Enchiridion* for modern times. He's done a truly incredible job and will no doubt go down in history as one of the great Stoic thinkers of our time. You should definitely check out this book. Especially if you're a fan of Epictetus.

Irvine, William B. *A Guide to the Good Life: The Ancient Art of Stoic Joy.* **OUP USA, 2009**
William has a beautiful way of writing and I absolutely love this book. It's a thorough and comprehensive guide to Stoicism and one of the finest books out there. I'm confident that you are going to get a lot out of this one.

Irvine, William B. *The Stoic Challenge: A Philosopher's Guide to Becoming Tougher, Calmer and More Resilient.* **WW Norton & Co, 2019**
This book focuses on dealing with setbacks and reframing difficulty as a challenge. It's very practical and gets you to test

out ideas in the real world. If you've enjoyed my book, I think you'll find this helpful and engaging too.

Holiday, Ryan. *The Obstacle is the Way: The Ancient Art of Turning Adversity to Advantage.* Profile Books, 2015
This is a brilliant book that has been the gateway into Stoicism for a lot of people. It's become a bit of a cult classic and really helped to put Stoicism on the map. The book focuses on the ability to handle obstacles and setbacks with grace and finesse, just like the Stoics.

Goodman, Rob. *Rome's Last Citizen: The Life and Legacy of Cato, Mortal Enemy of Caesar.* Griffin, 2014
This book is a well-researched and fascinating look at the life of Cato. It will give you an insight into how this Stoic lived his life and share with you some really interesting stories. This is brilliant for those keen to learn more about the history of the Stoics.

Hadot, Pierre. *The Inner Citadel: The Meditations of Marcus Aurelius.* Harvard University Press, 2001
If you want to get into the nitty gritty details of Marcus Aurelius' life and philosophy, then this is the book for you. It's a little on the academic side of things, but that is exactly what we want if we are going to look at things in real depth. It's an important book in the Stoic community and you will likely get Stoic bonus points for knowing about this one.

WIDER/FURTHER READING SUGGESTIONS

After working through the previous list of Stoic books, you might want to consider taking things a little further. In this section, I've branched out and given some recommendations for philosophy in general. I've also included all of the books I have mentioned earlier in my writing. Some of these have a tenuous link to Stoicism, but I believe that they will complement your Stoic library well.

Edgley, Ross. *The Art of Resilience*. HarperCollins, 2020
This book is truly inspirational. It documents Ross' world record swim around Great Britain and will get you fired up in search of your own epic challenges. The book is threaded with Stoic philosophy and there are plenty of practical ideas to take away from it. Ross is a fantastic example of a "modern Stoic" – he is both humble and hardworking and you can't help but feel motivated after working through these pages. It's a wonderful read and shows someone using Stoicism to achieve extraordinary things in the modern world.

Frank, Anne. *The Diary of a Young Girl: The Definitive Edition of the World's Most Famous Diary*. Penguin, 2012
It's hard to read this book and not be deeply moved by Anne's words and experiences. It shows the power of the diary and what a wonderful tool a journal can be. I can't recommend it enough.

Itzler, Jesse. *Living with a SEAL: 31 Days Training with the Toughest Man on the Planet*. Center Street, 2017
As mentioned earlier, this is a great example of voluntary discomfort in the modern world. Having a Navy SEAL live with

you is a pretty extreme way to practise this idea, but it makes for a wonderfully entertaining read.

Cathcart, Thomas and Klein, Daniel. *Plato and a Platypus Walk into a Bar ... Understanding Philosophy Through Jokes.* Penguin Books, 2008
If you want to learn more about philosophy in a fun and accessible way, this is the book for you! It's got tons of jokes in it and will keep you smiling while you read it. I highly recommend it.

Cathcart, Thomas and Klein, Daniel. *Heidegger and a Hippo Walk Through Those Pearly Gates: Using Philosophy (and Jokes!) to Explore Life, Death, the Afterlife, and Everything in Between.* Penguin USA, 2011
Witty, sharp and highly amusing, the second book that merges comedy and philosophy from Daniel Klein and Thomas Cathcart is just as brilliant as the first. It's a quick read but packed with wisdom from a variety of different sources.

Evans, Jules. *Philosophy for Life: And Other Dangerous Situations.* Rider, 2013
There's a great section on Stoicism in this fantastic book, but it also takes a further look at other philosophy in general. It's a great place to start branching away from Stoicism and seeing what else is out there in the world of philosophy.

Russell, Bertrand. *History of Western Philosophy.* Routledge, 2004
This brick of a book has got you covered for all things philosophical. From the Socratic era, up to modern day, you will have a scholarly explanation of it all. It's hands down one of the most important philosophical works of all time and does an incredible job of putting Western philosophy in one place.

If you study philosophy at university, this is one of the essential books on the reading list.

Macaro, Antonia. *More Than Happiness: Buddhist and Stoic Wisdom for a Sceptical Age*. Icon Books Ltd, 2018

This book is a direct comparison of Buddhism and Stoicism – it's amazing how many similarities there are! Antonia does a wonderful job of highlighting this and I think you'll really enjoy it.

Wright, Robert. *Why Buddhism is True: The Science and Philosophy of Meditation and Enlightenment*. Simon & Schuster, 2018

This is one of my favourite books on Buddhism. It's so beautifully written and looks at things through the eyes of evolutionary science. It's fascinating! You'll notice some real similarities to Stoicism here and I think it's interesting to be aware of this.

Harris, Russ. *The Happiness Trap: Stop Struggling, Start Living*. Robinson Publishing, 2008

If you want to further your understanding of ACT (mentioned earlier in this book), you need not search any further. This is brilliant for those wanting to explore the therapy in detail. It's really well written and will be particularly helpful for those dealing with negative internal dialogue.

Wilding, Christine. *Cognitive Behavioural Therapy*. Teach Yourself, 2015

This is a great book for looking deeper into CBT. It's highly accessible and will get you blasting all of your negative thoughts with logic in no time at all!

ONLINE STOIC RESOURCES

There are so many wonderful places where you can get your Stoic fix online and tons of YouTube videos, podcasts, blogposts and social media accounts for you to explore. Some of them are better than others. And some are a LOT better than others. Rather than overwhelm you with choices, I would like to recommend the following two websites as a solid place to start. These are my favourite sites and should keep you busy for a while:

www.modernstoicism.com
www.dailystoic.com

THE STOIC CHEAT SHEET

Think of this section as a quick recap and guide to ideas and technical words from Stoic philosophy. I've only included stuff that I've mentioned in the book – so don't worry, it's not a long list of random things.

EUDAIMONIA
The purpose of Stoicism. Essentially – happiness/tranquillity/balance/flourishing/wellbeing.

ARETÊ
To be the best version of ourselves in every moment.

INDIFFERENCES
These are things which are neither intrinsically good or bad, as they are typically outside of our control (for the most part). Examples are money, reputation, health, looks, etc.

PREFERRED INDIFFERENCES
Things that are technically indifferent, but we would prefer them if we had a choice: e.g. good health, or a fat wedge of cash.

THE CARDINAL VIRTUES
The classic virtues that the Stoics would use as guidance: Fortitude, Wisdom, Justice and Temperance. You remember the example of the wig-wearing, self-disciplined lion, right?!

OIKEIÔSIS
Bringing others closer to you. Not literally, but more like appropriating – making part of you. Caring for strangers as if

they were part of the family. Not treating Susie like an outcast at Christmas. That sort of thing.

PROSOCHĒ
Attention/mindfulness. This is the awareness we should strive to bring to our own behaviour. Similar to being present – but focused on how the mind is in that moment.

APATHEIA
Being able to control our emotions and not get caught up in them. This is not the suppression of emotions, but the ability to remain in control of them.

PROPATHEIAI
Our initial reactions. For example – if someone scares us, we jump with surprise. Totally normal.

SYMPATHEIA
The interconnectedness of all of humanity, nature and the universe.

PASSIONS
Essentially strong negative emotions.

STOA POIKILE
The giant arch/porch/building thing in the north of Athens where Zeno and all of the other Greek heads of Stoicism would lecture.

THE DICHOTOMY OF CONTROL/THE STOIC GOLDEN RULE
We can't control external events, but we can choose how we respond to them.

LIVING IN AGREEMENT WITH NATURE
Using logic and reasoning as guiding principles.

HUPEXAIRESIS
Also known as The Stoic Reserve Clause, this is essentially the process of reminding ourselves that nothing is guaranteed. It's similar to tagging "fate permitting" on to the end of our sentences about future plans.

DISCIPLINE OF ASSENT
This is the application of logic and reasoning to the way we live our lives. The ability to stay in control when facing tough emotions and make informed judgements.

DISCIPLINE OF ACTION
This is based on Stoic ethics and focuses on our behaviour. It also looks at our relationship with the rest of humanity.

DISCIPLINE OF DESIRE
This discipline looks at what we can and can't control and encourages us to think about the cosmic order of things.

AMOR FATI
A love of fate – essentially the ability to embrace whatever happens to us.

MEMENTO MORI
This is a Latin phrase meaning "remember you are mortal".

ASKÊSIS
The Stoic word for training.

DATES OF THE STOICS

Below is a cast list of the main Stoics featured in this book and their respective dates. These will be handy if you have a dinner party to go to and want to get all fancy with philosophical dates:

- Zeno of Citium – 334–262 BCE
- Cleanthes – 330–230 BCE
- Chrysippus – 279–206 BCE
- Cato – 95–46 BCE
- Lucius Annaeus Seneca – 4 BCE–65 CE
- Musonius Rufus – 20/30–101 CE
- Epictetus – 55–135 CE
- Marcus Aurelius – 121–180 CE

THE STOIC PRINCIPLES

And a quick recap of the 10 game-changing ideas mentioned in this book:

1. VOLUNTARY DISCOMFORT
By deliberately stepping outside of our comfort zones and enduring discomfort in a host of different ways, we build resilience.

2. PERCEPTION
Our judgements of external events can have a huge impact on how we live our lives. We should pay attention to how our mind perceives the outside world and be conscious of our internal dialogue.

3. SETBACKS

When facing a setback, we need to ensure that we have the right mindset. We should focus on what we can control in the situation (rather than what we can't) and put our attention to good use by focusing on our response to everything.

4. SELF-REFLECTION

By examining our lives on a daily basis, we become more well-rounded individuals. We will also become aware of what areas in our lives need work as inward reflection can help us to understand ourselves better.

5. ROLE MODELS

We should seek out positive and negative role models in life. If we look at their behaviour, we can use this as inspiration for what to do or not to do.

6. NEGATIVE VISUALIZATION

If we think about what could go wrong, we can pre-emptively prepare for it happening in the future. We can also contemplate loss as a way to increase our gratitude for everything in our lives.

7. MANAGING STRONG EMOTIONS

When dealing with powerful negative emotions, we would be wise to insert a wedge of time before responding. Having a measured response to external events and the ability to be in control of our emotions is an important skill.

8. DEALING WITH OTHERS

We will likely encounter difficult people out there in the real world, but we can choose how we respond to this. We can turn a negative encounter into a test of character by focusing on how we manage the situation. We also need to remember that we are human beings and should focus on our common humanity when dealing with particularly tricky people.

9. MEMENTO MORI

By contemplating our mortality, we have a greater appreciation for life itself. This can help us to live with purpose, gratitude and direction.

10. THE COSMIC PERSPECTIVE

If we zoom out, we become aware of how brief our lives actually are. In the scheme of things, we don't have a lot of time. We would be wise to spend it carefully. Actively engaging with nature and the community helps us to develop a deeper connection with everything around us.

ACKNOWLEDGEMENTS

I'd like to thank the following people for helping me with this project:

My brilliant publishers – Welbeck Publishing. It's been a lovely experience working with them and I've had the pleasure of collaborating with so many talented people along the way. I'd like to deeply thank everyone at Welbeck involved in bringing this book together. Thank you! I really appreciate all of your hard work.

My agent Robert Gwyn Palmer has been the voice of reason and support since day one. It's been exciting to bring out another book and I've been very appreciative of Robert's continual sage advice throughout this process. It's been an honour for me to have him in my corner.

Jo Lal has had a humungous influence on this book and I'm so grateful for all of her wisdom and input. Without her, none of this would have been possible. I feel incredibly lucky that I've been able to work with her again. She is truly magnificent at what she does and has helped to shape this project into something that I am extremely proud of and excited to be sharing with the world.

Kate Latham has been a wonderful editor to collaborate with on this book and I've absolutely loved working with her. Having joined forces together on my first book, I was delighted that we could be reunited again for this project. She is a true professional and I've learned so much from her.

My friends have been devout supporters of my writing and I'm incredibly grateful for all of them. Whether it's deep philosophical chats, spicy climbs, cold dips or just good old honest hanging out and being silly, I'm a lucky man to have so many wonderful people in my life that support me so much. Thank you all – you know who you are!

Special thanks go to my mum and dad for their continual feedback on this project. I really appreciate everything that they have done and the amount of time they have invested in reading my work. You are a pair of legends!

And then we have Helen. My Stoic wife. I'm continually blown away by the level of support that she offers me. Even when I'm doing something ridiculous like climbing Everest on my stairs, she's there cheering me on. It means the world to me and I will be forever grateful for having her in my life. She also happens to be a wonderful proofreader and has helped me so much with her wise feedback and ideas on this book. So, extra bonus points there!

And finally, I would like to say a massive thank you to you. Yes, you! As a reader of this book you are helping me realize my dream of being a writer. Without you, I would just be talking to myself. Thank you for coming on this journey with me. I really appreciate your support.

COME AND SAY HI

One of the best things about putting my first book out into the world was hearing from readers. It's lovely to connect with you all so do come and let me know how you're getting on with everything. Don't be shy!

I'm most active on Instagram but you'll also find me on Twitter. My website has a ton of resources too. And if you're keen to stay up to date with my current and future projects, I put out a monthly newsletter. This has book recommendations, quotes and links to media appearances – blog posts/articles/podcasts, etc. You can sign up for this on my website. Don't worry, it's not spammy! Quality over quantity is my ethos.

⊙ @dothingsthatchallengeyou
🐦 @iambenaldridge
🌐 www.benaldridge.com
   (sign up found at the bottom of each page)

I'm asked a lot to talk about Stoic philosophy in corporate and business settings, so please feel free to reach out if you're ever in need of Stoic training in the workplace. I absolutely love exploring how Stoicism can bring resilience and positivity to different teams.

I look forward to meeting you either in the virtual or real world!

TriggerHub.org is one of the most elite and scientifically proven forms of mental health intervention

Trigger Publishing is the leading independent mental health and wellbeing publisher in the UK and US. Clinical and scientific research conducted by assistant professor Dr Kristin Kosyluk and her highly acclaimed team in the Department of Mental Health Law & Policy at the University of South Florida (USF), as well as complementary research by her peers across the US, has independently verified the power of lived experience as a core component in achieving mental health prosperity. Specifically, the lived experiences contained within our bibliotherapeutic books are intrinsic elements in reducing stigma, making those with poor mental health feel less alone, providing the privacy they need to heal, ensuring they know the essential steps to kick-start their own journeys to recovery, and providing hope and inspiration when they need it most.

Delivered through TriggerHub, our unique online portal and accompanying smartphone app, we make our library of bibliotherapeutic titles and other vital resources accessible to individuals and organizations anywhere, at any time and with complete privacy, a crucial element of recovery. As such, TriggerHub is the primary recommendation across the UK and US for the delivery of lived experiences.

At Trigger Publishing and TriggerHub, we proudly lead the way in making the unseen become seen. We are dedicated to humanizing mental health, breaking stigma and challenging outdated societal values to create real action and impact. Find out more about our world-leading work with lived experience and bibliotherapy via triggerhub.org, or by joining us on:

🐦 @triggerhub_

⬤ @triggerhub.org

◉ @triggerhub_